The Glutathione Reset

How Your Body Loses Energy, Builds Toxins, and Breaks Down And How to Restore It

First Edition: March 2026
ISBN: 978-1-966035-05-3
Published by Elite Nutrition Research
EliteNutritionResearch.com

ELITE

NUTRITION RESEARCH

Elite Nutrition Research is a science-driven health and education company dedicated to understanding and optimizing human physiology at its most fundamental level. Our work is built on an architecture-first approach—examining how nutrients interact with cellular systems, membranes, energy production, and signaling pathways to shape overall health and performance. Rather than following trends, we focus on first principles, combining biochemical insight, formulation precision, and practical application to create both advanced nutritional products and in-depth educational systems.

Through our books, courses, and formulations, Elite Nutrition Research aims to give individuals direct access to the mechanisms that govern their biology empowering them to think clearly, act intentionally, and build lasting health from the inside out.

To explore our full system of products, courses, and research, visit:
www.elitenutritionresearch.com

Table of Contents

The modern environment increases the demand placed on this system while simultaneously constraining its inputs. Chemical exposure, processed food intake, disrupted sleep, and chronic stress all increase reactive load or reduce the availability of the substrates required to maintain glutathione. The result is not an immediate collapse but a gradual loss of completion capacity. Reactions continue to occur, but fewer of them are fully resolved. Over time, this leads to accumulation of damaged molecules, impaired signaling, and reduced energy efficiency. The system becomes unstable, not because it lacks activity, but because it cannot finish what it starts.

Glutathione should not be viewed as a supplementable endpoint or a single lever that can be pulled to restore health. It reflects the state of a larger network that includes amino acid availability, mitochondrial function, enzymatic capacity, and cellular organization. Increasing glutathione without addressing these underlying factors produces limited and temporary effects because the system that sustains it remains unchanged. Restoration requires rebuilding the conditions that allow glutathione to be continuously synthesized, recycled, and distributed across cellular compartments.

When this system is intact, the cell operates with precision. Reactive intermediates are contained, energy production remains stable, signaling pathways function within defined limits, and external compounds are processed and removed without accumulation. When it is impaired, instability appears across multiple systems at once. Energy becomes inconsistent, inflammation persists, detoxification slows, and structural damage accumulates. These outcomes are often treated as separate problems, but they share a common origin in the loss of redox control. Glutathione does not act as a peripheral support molecule. It defines whether the internal environment remains ordered under load or degrades as demand increases.

Glutathione as a Threshold Molecule for Survival

Glutathione functions as a boundary condition that determines whether cellular processes remain contained or begin to destabilize the structures that support them. Every cell operates under continuous chemical flux, generating reactive intermediates through energy production, substrate transformation, and environmental exposure. These intermediates are not inherently pathological, but they require immediate handling to prevent interaction with proteins, lipids, and nucleic acids. Glutathione provides the primary buffering capacity that absorbs this reactivity and returns it to a controlled state. As long as intracellular levels remain above a critical range, the cell can complete these reactions without structural loss. When levels fall below that range, the same reactions begin to produce cumulative damage, not because the processes themselves change, but because their byproducts are no longer contained.

This threshold is not defined by a single concentration value but by the relationship between reduced and oxidized glutathione within specific cellular compartments. The ratio between these forms determines the redox environment that proteins operate within. Many enzymes rely on thiol groups that must remain in a reduced state to maintain proper structure and function. As oxidized glutathione accumulates, these thiol groups form disulfide bonds, altering protein configuration and reducing enzymatic activity. This shift propagates through metabolic pathways, slowing reactions that depend on precise protein geometry. The cell begins to lose efficiency, and processes that were previously self-contained start to leak reactive intermediates into surrounding systems.

Mitochondria operate closest to this threshold due to their continuous production of reactive oxygen species during electron transport. Under stable conditions, glutathione neutralizes these species as they are formed, preventing interaction with mitochondrial membranes and DNA. When glutathione availability drops, reactive species escape containment and initiate lipid peroxidation within the inner mitochondrial membrane. This alters membrane integrity and disrupts electron flow, reducing ATP production while increasing further reactive output. The system enters a feedback loop where declining energy production increases instability, which in turn accelerates oxidative damage.

Detoxification pathways exhibit the same dependence on threshold conditions. Phase I reactions introduce reactive groups into compounds to prepare them for removal, but without sufficient glutathione, these intermediates persist in a chemically active state. Instead of being conjugated and eliminated, they interact with cellular structures or circulate back through the system. The detoxification process becomes incomplete, increasing total reactive load rather than reducing it. The cell is then forced to allocate additional resources to manage these unresolved intermediates, further straining glutathione reserves.

Immune activity places intermittent but intense demand on this system. During activation, immune cells generate reactive species to disrupt pathogens. Resolution requires a rapid restoration of redox balance to prevent collateral damage. When glutathione levels are sufficient, this transition occurs efficiently, and tissue integrity is preserved. When levels are below threshold, reactive species continue to be produced in an environment that cannot neutralize them effectively. The result is prolonged inflammation, where the immune response remains active but loses precision, damaging host tissue alongside its intended targets.

The concept of a threshold becomes clear when observing how quickly function deteriorates once glutathione falls below a certain capacity. Above this level, the system maintains stability despite fluctuations in demand. Below it, small increases in reactive load produce disproportionate effects, as the buffering system can no longer absorb additional stress. This is not a gradual decline but a shift in system behavior. The cell transitions from controlled processing to progressive disruption, where damage accumulates faster than it can be repaired.

Restoring this threshold requires more than increasing glutathione directly. The system must be supplied with the substrates, enzymatic activity, and reducing power needed to sustain continuous turnover. Without these inputs, any increase is temporary, and the cell remains near the boundary where instability can re-emerge. When the threshold is re-established and maintained, cellular processes return to a state where reactions are completed, intermediates are contained, and structural integrity is preserved under ongoing demand.

Cellular Resilience as a Function of Redox Completion

Cellular resilience is determined by whether chemical reactions are brought to completion without leaving reactive intermediates embedded in the system. Every metabolic event produces transitional states that carry excess electrons or unstable bonds. These states are necessary for transformation, but they cannot persist. If they remain unresolved, they begin to interact with nearby structures, modifying proteins, initiating lipid peroxidation, and altering signaling pathways. Resilience emerges when the cell can process these intermediates fully, returning them to stable end products while preserving the integrity of surrounding components. This capacity is governed by the redox environment, which defines how efficiently electrons are transferred, neutralized, and redistributed across the system.

Glutathione provides the central mechanism for completing these reactions because it can accept and donate electrons in a controlled and reversible manner. Its reduced form absorbs oxidative load, and its oxidized form is returned to a usable state through enzymatic recycling that depends on NADPH. This continuous cycle allows the cell to manage a steady influx of reactive intermediates without accumulating damage. When this system operates within capacity, reactions proceed in sequence and terminate cleanly. Substrates are converted, energy is extracted, and byproducts are either neutralized or removed. The cell maintains structural coherence because each step in the process is followed by a resolution phase that restores chemical stability.

When redox completion begins to fail, the sequence breaks. Intermediates are generated faster than they can be neutralized, and partially reacted molecules persist within the intracellular environment. Proteins with exposed thiol groups become oxidized and shift configuration, reducing catalytic efficiency. Lipid membranes begin to incorporate oxidized fatty acids, altering fluidity and permeability. Signaling pathways that depend on controlled redox states become distorted, producing either prolonged activation or insufficient response. The system does not stop functioning, but it operates in a degraded mode where each reaction contributes additional instability instead of resolving it.

Mitochondria illustrate this dependence on completion with high sensitivity. Electron transport relies on precise handoff of electrons across complexes embedded in the inner membrane. When glutathione and associated systems maintain redox balance, electrons move efficiently toward oxygen, and ATP production remains stable. When redox completion is impaired, electrons escape prematurely and react with oxygen to form reactive species that damage mitochondrial components. This reduces energy output while increasing the burden of reactive intermediates, forcing the cell to operate with less energy while managing greater instability. The mismatch between production and containment drives further dysfunction.

Detoxification pathways follow the same principle. The initial modification of compounds increases their reactivity to prepare them for conjugation. Without sufficient redox capacity, these intermediates accumulate and interact with cellular structures instead of being neutralized. Glutathione conjugation represents the completion step that renders these compounds transportable and removable. If this step is delayed or insufficient, the system retains partially processed molecules that continue to generate reactive stress. Detoxification becomes an incomplete loop, increasing internal load rather than clearing it.

Immune responses depend on controlled disruption followed by completion. Reactive species are generated to damage pathogens, but this must be followed by rapid restoration of a reduced intracellular environment to prevent collateral damage. When glutathione and its supporting systems are sufficient, the transition from activation to resolution occurs with precision. When they are limited, the system remains in a partially activated state, where reactive molecules continue to circulate without effective containment. This prolongs inflammation and extends damage beyond the initial target.

Resilience, in this context, is not defined by the absence of stress but by the ability to finish the chemical processes that stress initiates. A resilient cell can tolerate high levels of metabolic activity, environmental exposure, and immune activation because it maintains the capacity to resolve the intermediates these processes generate. When redox completion is intact, the system absorbs variability without structural degradation. When it is compromised, even moderate inputs produce cumulative damage because reactions remain open-ended. The difference between stability and breakdown is determined by whether the cell can close these loops consistently over time.

Modern Overload vs Declining Capacity

The current environment increases the number of reactions the body must process while reducing the resources required to complete them. This mismatch is not abstract. It is mechanical. Every exposure introduces substrates that must be transformed, neutralized, or removed, and each of those steps generates intermediate states that require containment. Chemical inputs from food additives, environmental compounds, and metabolic byproducts all enter processing pathways that depend on redox balance. At the same time, dietary patterns often reduce the intake of amino acids and micronutrients required to sustain glutathione synthesis and recycling. The system is pushed to operate at higher throughput while its capacity to resolve intermediates is constrained.

Mitochondria carry a large share of this increased demand because energy production must scale with environmental and physiological stress. Higher throughput through the electron transport chain increases the probability of electron leakage, producing reactive species that must be neutralized immediately. When glutathione availability and recycling capacity are sufficient, this increased flux remains contained. When they are limited, reactive output exceeds buffering capacity and begins to interact with mitochondrial membranes and proteins. Energy production becomes less efficient, which forces the system to push even more substrate through the same pathways to maintain output. This creates a cycle where declining efficiency increases reactive load, further reducing capacity.

Detoxification pathways show the same imbalance. The number and diversity of compounds requiring processing has increased, but the capacity for conjugation and elimination has not scaled accordingly. Phase I reactions continue to introduce reactive groups into these compounds, but without sufficient glutathione, the conjugation step is delayed or incomplete. Intermediates remain active, circulating through tissues and interacting with cellular structures. Instead of being removed, they add to the total reactive burden. Each incomplete cycle increases the demand placed on an already constrained system.

Nutrient availability plays a direct role in this decline. Glutathione synthesis depends on cysteine, glycine, and glutamate, along with enzymatic activity that requires adequate micronutrient support. Diets that reduce protein intake or rely on processed foods often fail to supply these components in sufficient quantities. At the same time, chronic stress alters metabolism in a way that prioritizes immediate energy production over maintenance functions such as antioxidant recycling. NADPH availability can become limited, reducing the rate at which oxidized glutathione is returned to its functional state. The system loses both input and recycling efficiency simultaneously.

Immune activation further amplifies this imbalance. Persistent low-level stimulation from environmental and metabolic stressors keeps the immune system in a semi-active state, producing reactive molecules that must be neutralized even in the absence of acute infection. When glutathione capacity is intact, these responses resolve quickly and do not accumulate. When capacity is reduced, the system remains partially activated, generating a continuous background level of reactive species that consume available resources without reaching resolution. This ongoing demand prevents recovery and maintains the system in a state of incomplete processing.

The interaction between increased demand and reduced capacity creates a shift in system behavior. Under balanced conditions, the body processes inputs, neutralizes intermediates, and restores baseline stability. Under modern conditions, inputs exceed the rate at which they can be resolved. Intermediates accumulate, reactions remain open, and structural damage begins to outpace repair. The system does not fail immediately. It transitions into a state where each additional demand produces a larger effect because the buffering capacity has been eroded.

Restoring stability requires more than reducing exposure or increasing a single input. The system must be rebuilt so that throughput and completion capacity are aligned again. This means increasing substrate availability for glutathione synthesis, restoring enzymatic and recycling efficiency, and reducing unnecessary reactive load where possible. When capacity is restored, the same environment produces less disruption because the system can process and complete reactions without accumulation. When capacity remains constrained, even moderate inputs continue to push the system beyond its ability to resolve them.

Reframing Disease as Loss of Completion Capacity

Disease can be understood as the point at which biological processes continue to initiate but fail to resolve. The body does not stop reacting to inputs. It continues to generate energy, process substrates, activate immune responses, and attempt detoxification. The breakdown occurs in the closing phase of these processes, where reactive intermediates are meant to be neutralized, transformed, and cleared. When completion fails, these intermediates persist within the system and begin interacting with structures that were not part of the original reaction. Proteins become modified, membranes incorporate damaged lipids, and signaling pathways shift away from controlled regulation toward prolonged activation. What is often labeled as separate disease states emerges from this shared condition of incomplete processing.

At the molecular level, this failure is expressed through disruption of redox balance. Glutathione-dependent systems lose the ability to maintain a reduced environment, and the ratio between reduced and oxidized forms shifts toward an oxidized state. This change alters the behavior of proteins that rely on thiol groups for structural integrity and catalytic activity. Enzymes slow or misfire, transport systems lose selectivity, and regulatory proteins that depend on redox-sensitive switches begin to send distorted signals. The system becomes less precise. Reactions that once followed defined pathways begin to diverge, producing side products that further increase the burden on an already constrained network.

Inflammation illustrates this pattern with clarity. An immune response is initiated to address a specific challenge, generating reactive species and signaling molecules that disrupt the target. Completion requires that this response be contained and resolved once the objective is achieved. When glutathione capacity is sufficient, the intracellular environment shifts back toward a reduced state, inflammatory signaling decreases, and tissue repair proceeds. When capacity is limited, the system cannot transition out of the activated state. Reactive molecules continue to circulate, and signaling pathways remain engaged. The result is chronic

Chapter 1

Early Discovery of Glutathione

Glutathione entered the scientific record before there was a framework capable of explaining what it was doing. Early biochemical work identified it as a sulfur-containing compound present within cells, but the context required to interpret its role did not yet exist. At the time, metabolism was being mapped in fragments, with individual reactions studied in isolation rather than as coordinated systems. Researchers could observe that glutathione was abundant in tissues and responsive to chemical conditions, but they lacked a model that connected those observations to a larger function. The molecule was cataloged, measured, and occasionally manipulated, yet its significance remained obscured because the systems it operated within had not been fully described.

Frederick Gowland Hopkins and other early investigators recognized that certain small molecules were essential for maintaining cellular activity, even if they were not classified as primary nutrients or structural components. Glutathione was grouped into this category of intracellular factors that appeared necessary for normal function. Its ability to undergo reversible oxidation drew attention, as it behaved differently from compounds that were consumed in a single reaction. It could shift between reduced and oxidized states, suggesting participation in ongoing chemical processes rather than one-time transformations. This behavior was noted, but without a clear understanding of redox systems, it was treated as an interesting property rather than the basis of a central regulatory function.

Analytical limitations also shaped how glutathione was perceived. Techniques for measuring intracellular concentrations were crude by modern standards, and compartmental differences within the cell were largely inaccessible. Researchers worked with homogenized tissue samples, which obscured the distinct environments of the cytosol, mitochondria, and other organelles. Without the ability to see how glutathione was distributed or how its levels changed in specific locations, its role appeared diffuse and nonspecific. It was present everywhere, which made it difficult to assign to any single pathway. This led to the assumption that it was supportive rather than essential, a background molecule that assisted more important processes rather than defining them.

The conceptual gap was not due to a lack of observation but to the absence of a systems-level model. Oxidation and reduction were understood as chemical reactions, but their integration into cellular control mechanisms had not yet been articulated. The idea that a molecule could maintain a dynamic balance across multiple pathways, influencing enzyme activity, structural integrity, and signaling simultaneously, required a shift in how biology was organized. Early research operated within a framework that separated processes into discrete categories, which made it difficult to recognize a molecule that moved between them and influenced each one through a shared mechanism.

As biochemical methods improved, patterns began to emerge that hinted at a broader role. Changes in glutathione levels were associated with shifts in cellular stability, particularly under conditions of stress. Depletion correlated with increased susceptibility to damage, while restoration improved recovery. These observations accumulated across different tissues and experimental conditions, gradually building a case that glutathione was involved in maintaining internal balance. Even then, it was often described in narrow terms, linked to specific reactions or protective effects without integrating those functions into a unified system.

The early history of glutathione reflects a common pattern in biological discovery. A molecule is identified and characterized chemically before its role within the larger system is understood. The delay between discovery and recognition is not a failure of observation but a limitation of perspective. Without a model that connects structure to function across multiple levels, the significance of a molecule that operates at the intersection of those levels remains hidden. Glutathione was present, active, and essential long before it was understood, functioning as part of a system that science had not yet learned to describe.

Initial Identification as a Sulfur Compound

Glutathione was first recognized through its sulfur content, not through an understanding of its role in cellular systems. Early biochemical analysis focused on isolating compounds from tissue extracts and classifying them based on elemental composition and reactivity. Sulfur-containing molecules attracted attention because sulfur exhibited distinct chemical behavior, particularly its ability to participate in reversible oxidation and form stable yet reactive bonds. When glutathione was identified within cells, it was grouped with other sulfur compounds, defined primarily by the presence of a reactive thiol group rather than by any clear functional integration into metabolism.

The methods used at the time shaped this interpretation. Tissue samples were homogenized and subjected to chemical separation techniques that could detect functional groups but could not preserve spatial organization or dynamic activity. Glutathione appeared as a small, soluble molecule with a sulfhydryl group that reacted predictably under oxidizing conditions. Researchers could observe that it shifted between reduced and oxidized states, forming disulfide bonds when exposed to oxidative environments. This behavior distinguished it from many other intracellular compounds, but without a framework for redox systems, it was treated as a chemical curiosity rather than a central feature of cellular regulation.

Sulfur chemistry itself provided clues that were not fully developed at the time. The thiol group on cysteine carries a high capacity for electron exchange, allowing it to interact with reactive species in a controlled manner. When glutathione was oxidized, two molecules linked through a disulfide bond, and this bond could be reversed under reducing conditions. This reversibility implied a cycle rather than a one-directional reaction. The molecule could absorb oxidative load and then be restored to its original state, suggesting a role in maintaining chemical balance. Early researchers documented these transformations, but they lacked the conceptual link that connected this behavior to broader cellular stability.

The classification of glutathione as a sulfur compound also limited how it was studied. It was compared to other thiol-containing molecules and evaluated within that narrow category, which emphasized chemical properties over system-level function. This approach separated it from pathways involving energy production, detoxification, and signaling, even though its behavior directly influenced each of those processes. By focusing on composition rather than integration, early work placed glutathione at the periphery of biochemical models instead of at their center.

Despite these limitations, certain observations pointed toward a larger role. Glutathione was found in high concentrations across many tissues, a pattern that did not align with a minor or specialized function. Its levels changed in response to environmental conditions, particularly those that increased oxidative stress. These shifts indicated that it was not static but actively involved in responding to changes within the cellular environment. The sulfur group that defined its classification was also the feature that enabled this responsiveness, allowing it to interact with reactive intermediates and influence the outcome of ongoing reactions.

The initial identification of glutathione as a sulfur compound established the foundation for understanding its chemical capabilities, but it did not capture its position within the system. The focus on sulfur highlighted its reactivity and reversibility, yet the absence of a systems-level model prevented those properties from being recognized as central to cellular control. What appeared as a defining characteristic at the chemical level was only one part of a larger architecture, where that reactivity would later be understood as the mechanism through which the cell maintains stability under continuous metabolic activity.Hopkins and early biochemical context

Why Its Importance Was Missed

Glutathione was identified early, measured repeatedly, and shown to change under stress, yet it remained peripheral in biological models because it did not fit into the way metabolism was organized at the time. Early biochemistry separated processes into discrete pathways with defined inputs and outputs, favoring molecules that could be assigned to a single reaction or a clearly bounded sequence. Glutathione did not behave that way. It moved across pathways, participated in multiple reactions, and cycled between states without being consumed. This made it difficult to classify. It did not present as a substrate, a product, or a conventional cofactor, so it was treated as supportive rather than structural to the system.

The dominant framework focused on linear reactions where cause and effect could be traced step by step. In that context, importance was assigned to molecules that produced visible changes when added or removed. Glutathione did not produce a single defining effect. Instead, it altered the conditions under which many reactions occurred. It influenced enzyme activity, stabilized proteins, and buffered reactive intermediates, but these effects were distributed and conditional. When present at sufficient levels, processes appeared normal and required no explanation. Only when it declined did dysfunction emerge, and even then, the resulting changes were spread across multiple systems, making it difficult to attribute them to a single cause.

Analytical limitations reinforced this misinterpretation. Measurements were taken from homogenized tissues, which removed the spatial organization that defines cellular function. Glutathione appeared uniformly present, obscuring the fact that its role varies by compartment and that local depletion can have system-wide effects. Without the ability to observe these gradients, researchers saw abundance without specificity. A molecule that is everywhere can appear unimportant because its absence is rarely isolated to a single observable change. The tools available at the time could detect concentration but not functional distribution.

The concept of redox balance itself was underdeveloped. Oxidation and reduction were understood as chemical events, but their integration into cellular control systems had not yet been established. Without a model that connected electron flow to enzyme behavior, membrane integrity, and signaling, glutathione's cycling between reduced and oxidized states was seen as a property rather than a function. The idea that a molecule could maintain system stability by managing electron distribution across multiple pathways required a shift from reaction-based thinking to systems-based thinking. That shift had not yet occurred.

There was also a bias toward molecules that acted in a directional manner. Substrates are converted, hormones trigger responses, and enzymes catalyze specific reactions. Glutathione operates through reversibility and continuous turnover. It absorbs reactive load and is restored to its original state, allowing the process to repeat. This cyclical behavior does not produce a clear start and end point that can be easily measured. It maintains conditions rather than driving a single outcome. In a framework that prioritized directional causality, this made it appear secondary, even though it was defining whether those directional processes could proceed without disruption.

As research progressed and systems-level models began to form, the pattern became clearer. Glutathione was not acting on the system from the outside. It was maintaining the internal conditions that allowed the system to function. Its importance had been missed not because it was inactive or subtle, but because it operated at a level that earlier models were not designed to detect. Once biology began to account for compartmentalization, redox control, and network behavior, glutathione shifted from a background molecule to a central component of cellular stability.

Fragmented Observations Without System Model

Early research on glutathione produced a consistent pattern of findings that never converged into a coherent explanation because each observation was interpreted in isolation. Investigators measured its presence in tissues, documented its reversible oxidation, and noted that its levels changed under stress, but these results were treated as separate phenomena rather than components of a unified system. Without a framework that linked redox chemistry to cellular structure and function, glutathione appeared to participate in many unrelated processes instead of defining a common mechanism underlying them. The molecule was visible everywhere but understood nowhere because there was no model to integrate its behavior across compartments and pathways.

This fragmentation was reinforced by the way experiments were designed. Studies focused on single variables within controlled conditions, often removing glutathione from its native context to observe how it reacted in simplified systems. These approaches could demonstrate chemical properties, such as its ability to form disulfide bonds or interact with reactive species, but they stripped away the spatial organization and dynamic flux that give those properties meaning inside a living cell. When results from these experiments were brought back into biological interpretation, they were attached to specific reactions or pathways rather than recognized as part of a broader regulatory network. Each finding added detail without building structure.

The absence of a system model also meant that relationships between observations were missed. Changes in glutathione levels during oxidative stress were documented, but the connection between those changes and enzyme function, membrane stability, or signaling behavior was not fully developed. Researchers could see correlations but lacked the conceptual tools to trace cause and effect across multiple layers of organization. A decline in glutathione might be linked to increased cellular damage in one study and to altered detoxification in another, yet these outcomes were not unified under a single mechanism. They remained as separate lines of evidence pointing in the same direction without being connected.

Compartmentalization further complicated interpretation. Glutathione operates differently in the cytosol, mitochondria, and other cellular regions, but early methods could not resolve these differences. Measurements taken from whole-cell extracts averaged these environments into a single value, masking local depletion and localized stress responses. As a result, researchers saw fluctuations in overall concentration without understanding how those fluctuations translated into functional changes within specific parts of the cell. The system-level behavior, where disruption in one compartment propagates to others, remained hidden.

Conceptually, biology at the time emphasized pathways over networks. Processes were mapped as linear sequences with defined inputs and outputs, which made it difficult to place a molecule that moved between pathways and influenced their conditions simultaneously. Glutathione did not fit into a single pathway diagram. It interacted with many, altering their behavior through a shared mechanism of electron exchange. Without a network-based model, these interactions appeared scattered and secondary. The molecule was treated as a participant in multiple processes rather than as a factor that determined how those processes operated.

As more data accumulated, the limitations of this fragmented approach became apparent. The same molecule was repeatedly implicated in stability, protection, detoxification, and recovery, yet these roles were described independently. The missing element was not additional data but a shift in perspective that could organize these observations into a single framework. Once redox balance, compartmental organization, and system-wide regulation were considered together, the pieces aligned. What had been seen as unrelated effects could be understood as different expressions of the same underlying function. Glutathione was not acting in fragments. It was being observed through a fragmented lens.Chapter 2 — From Curiosity to Central Molecule (implied)

Transition from Isolated Chemistry to System Biology

The shift from isolated chemistry to system biology required a change in what counted as an explanation. Early work could describe reactions and identify molecules, but it treated each transformation as a closed event with defined inputs and outputs. This approach captured how individual reactions occurred, yet it could not account for how those reactions behaved when embedded in a living cell where thousands of processes run simultaneously and share intermediates. Glutathione did not fit within the earlier model because its function was not tied to a single reaction. It moved across processes, linking them through a common mechanism of electron transfer, and its effects became visible only when those processes were viewed together.

As biochemical methods improved, it became possible to observe patterns that extended beyond individual reactions. Changes in glutathione levels began to correlate with shifts in cellular stability across different systems, including energy production, detoxification, and immune activity. These correlations pointed toward a role that was not confined to one pathway but instead influenced the conditions under which multiple pathways operated. The focus began to move away from identifying what a molecule reacted with and toward understanding how it altered the behavior of the system as a whole. This required integrating chemical properties with spatial organization, recognizing that the same molecule could have different effects depending on where it was located and how it interacted with surrounding structures.

Compartmentalization provided a critical piece of this transition. The cell is not a uniform environment but a collection of distinct regions with specific conditions and demands. Glutathione pools in the cytosol, mitochondria, and nucleus operate under different constraints, and changes in one compartment can influence others through shared metabolites and signaling pathways. Recognizing these compartments allowed researchers to see that glutathione was not simply present throughout the cell but actively maintained in different locations to support specific functions. This spatial perspective transformed it from a general antioxidant into a regulator of localized environments.

The concept of redox balance also evolved during this period. Instead of viewing oxidation and reduction as isolated reactions, they were understood as part of a continuous flow of electrons that needed to be managed across the entire system. Glutathione became central to this understanding because it could accept and donate electrons repeatedly, linking multiple reactions into a coordinated network. Its cycling between reduced and oxidized forms provided a way to stabilize this flow, preventing accumulation of reactive intermediates and maintaining conditions that allowed enzymes and structural components to function properly. This reframed redox chemistry from a collection of reactions into a control system that influenced nearly every aspect of cellular behavior.

Network thinking replaced linear pathway models as researchers began to map how processes interacted. Instead of viewing metabolism as a series of independent routes, it was understood as an interconnected system where changes in one area could propagate through others.

Glutathione emerged as a key node within this network, not because it directed specific pathways, but because it maintained the environment required for those pathways to operate. Its role was conditional rather than directive. It determined whether reactions could proceed without disruption, rather than dictating which reactions would occur.

This transition did not introduce new properties to glutathione. It revealed how existing properties functioned within a larger context. The ability to undergo reversible oxidation, once seen as a chemical detail, became the basis for a system that managed reactive load across the cell. High intracellular concentrations, previously considered nonspecific, were recognized as necessary to maintain buffering capacity under continuous demand. Observations that had appeared fragmented began to align when placed within a framework that accounted for structure, location, and interaction.

System biology did not replace chemistry but reorganized it. It connected individual reactions into a coherent structure where molecules like glutathione could be understood in terms of how they sustain the conditions required for life. Within this framework, glutathione is not defined by the reactions it participates in but by the stability it provides to the system that contains those reactions.

Emergence of Oxidative Stress as a Concept

The concept of oxidative stress did not appear as a single discovery. It formed gradually as researchers began to recognize that reactive species were not rare byproducts but constant outputs of normal metabolism that required continuous control. Early work treated oxidation as a discrete chemical event, often associated with damage or exposure to external agents. Over time, it became clear that oxidation was embedded within core cellular processes, particularly in energy production where electron transfer is essential. As electrons move through the mitochondrial transport system, a fraction escapes and reacts with oxygen, forming reactive species that must be neutralized immediately to prevent interaction with surrounding structures.

This realization shifted attention from individual reactions to the balance between production and containment. Reactive species were no longer viewed solely as harmful agents but as inevitable intermediates generated by the cell itself. The problem was not their existence but the system's ability to manage them. When production remained within the capacity of buffering systems such as glutathione, these intermediates were absorbed and resolved without consequence. When production exceeded that capacity, they accumulated and began to modify proteins, lipids, and nucleic acids. Oxidative stress emerged as the condition where this balance tipped, defined by the persistence of reactive intermediates rather than their initial formation.

The role of glutathione became clearer within this framework because it provided a direct measure of the system's ability to maintain balance. Its reduced form acted as a reservoir for electrons, neutralizing reactive species as they were formed. Its oxidized form reflected the load that had been absorbed. The ratio between these states began to serve as an indicator of whether the system was operating within capacity or approaching instability. This ratio influenced enzyme behavior, membrane integrity, and signaling pathways, linking the abstract concept of oxidative stress to measurable changes in cellular function.

As the concept developed, it expanded beyond acute damage to include chronic conditions where reactive intermediates persist at lower levels over extended periods. This form of stress does not produce immediate structural failure but gradually alters system behavior. Enzymes lose efficiency, membranes incorporate oxidized lipids, and signaling pathways shift toward prolonged activation. The cumulative effect is a slow erosion of stability, where the system remains active but operates with reduced precision. This reframing connected oxidative stress to a wide range of conditions that previously lacked a unifying explanation.

The emergence of this concept also highlighted the importance of completion in biological processes. Reactive species are generated as part of normal function, but they must be neutralized or incorporated into stable end products. When this completion step is intact, oxidative events are contained within the system. When it is impaired, intermediates remain active and begin to propagate damage. Oxidative stress, in this sense, represents a failure of completion rather than an excess of initiation. The system continues to produce reactive species as it always has, but it loses the capacity to resolve them.

This shift in understanding integrated multiple lines of research into a single framework. Observations of cellular damage, enzyme dysfunction, and altered signaling could be traced back to the same underlying condition of unresolved reactivity. Glutathione moved from being one of many antioxidants to a central component of the system that defines whether oxidative processes remain controlled. The concept of oxidative stress provided the missing link that connected its chemical properties to its role in maintaining cellular stability under continuous metabolic activity.

Recognition of Intracellular Defense Systems

The recognition of intracellular defense systems emerged when it became clear that reactive intermediates were not occasional disruptions but constant outputs of normal cellular activity. Energy production, substrate transformation, and immune signaling all generate reactive species as part of their operation. These reactions cannot be eliminated because they are required for function, which means the cell must be equipped to manage them continuously. This shifted the focus from preventing reactive species to understanding how the cell contains and resolves them. Defense was no longer defined as a response to external threat but as a built-in capacity that operates alongside every metabolic process.

This realization led to the identification of coordinated systems rather than isolated molecules. Enzymes such as superoxide dismutase, catalase, and glutathione peroxidase were found to act in sequence, converting reactive species into less reactive forms that could be further processed or removed. These enzymes did not operate independently. Their activity depended on the availability of substrates and cofactors, as well as the surrounding redox environment. Glutathione emerged within this system as a central component because it provided the reducing equivalents required to complete these reactions. It did not replace enzymatic activity but enabled it, allowing reactive intermediates to be fully neutralized rather than partially transformed.

Compartmentalization refined this understanding by showing that defense systems are distributed according to local demand. The mitochondria, where electron transport generates a continuous stream of reactive species, maintain their own glutathione pool and associated enzymes to protect internal structures. The cytosol provides broader buffering capacity, stabilizing reactions that occur throughout the cell. Membranes rely on interactions between glutathione-dependent systems and lipid-soluble components to prevent structural degradation. Each compartment operates under different conditions, and defense systems are organized to match those conditions rather than being uniformly applied.

The concept of defense also expanded to include maintenance of protein structure and signaling fidelity. Reactive intermediates can alter thiol groups on proteins, changing their conformation and activity. Intracellular defense systems prevent these modifications from becoming permanent by maintaining a reduced environment that preserves protein function. This extends to signaling pathways, where redox-sensitive switches control activation and deactivation cycles. When the defense system is intact, these switches operate within defined limits. When it is compromised, signaling becomes prolonged or erratic, reflecting a loss of control over the conditions that govern these pathways.

Detoxification was incorporated into this framework as part of the same system rather than a separate function. Compounds introduced into the body are modified to increase their reactivity, which allows them to be conjugated and eliminated. Without sufficient glutathione and associated enzymes, these intermediates remain active and interact with cellular structures. The defense system must therefore manage both internally generated reactive species and those introduced from external sources. The distinction between endogenous and exogenous stress becomes less relevant than the capacity to process and complete these reactions.

The recognition of intracellular defense systems marked a transition from viewing protection as an external barrier to understanding it as an internal, continuous process. These systems do not activate only during periods of stress. They operate at all times, maintaining conditions that allow cellular processes to proceed without accumulation of damage. Glutathione sits within this architecture as a central mediator, linking enzymatic reactions, compartmental organization, and redox balance into a unified system. Its role becomes visible only when this system is viewed as a whole, where defense is defined not by isolated actions but by the ability to sustain stability under constant reactive load.

PART II

MOLECULAR STRUCTURE → CHEMICAL CAPABILITY

Why glutathione works at all

Chapter 3

The Tripeptide Architecture

Glutathione is built from three amino acids, but its function cannot be understood by listing those components. The arrangement of glutamate, cysteine, and glycine creates a molecule with specific chemical behavior that is not replicated by the same amino acids in isolation or in a different sequence. This structure determines how glutathione interacts with reactive intermediates, how it is preserved within the cell, and how it cycles between functional states. The moleculc is small enough to move freely through intracellular spaces, yet it carries a reactive center that can absorb and transfer electrons with precision. Its architecture allows it to operate continuously, not as a consumed substrate but as a reusable component of the system that maintains redox balance.

The glutamate residue forms the structural foundation of the molecule through a gamma-glutamyl linkage that differs from standard peptide bonds. This bond resists degradation by most intracellular peptidases, which typically recognize alpha-peptide linkages. As a result, glutathione remains intact in environments where other small peptides would be rapidly broken down. This stability is not incidental. It ensures that the molecule persists at high intracellular concentrations, maintaining a constant buffering capacity rather than fluctuating with transient changes in synthesis or degradation. The glutamate position anchors the molecule within the cellular environment, allowing it to function as a standing reservoir rather than a short-lived intermediate.

Cysteine provides the functional core of glutathione through its thiol group. This sulfur-containing site carries the capacity for reversible electron exchange, allowing glutathione to interact directly with reactive oxygen species and other electrophilic compounds. When the thiol group donates an electron, it becomes oxidized and forms a disulfide bond with another glutathione molecule. This conversion from reduced glutathione to its oxidized form represents the absorption of reactive load. The reaction is controlled and reversible, which allows the molecule to participate in ongoing cycles of oxidation and reduction without being permanently altered. The cysteine residue defines the molecule's ability to engage with reactive intermediates and determines how effectively those intermediates are contained.

Glycine completes the structure by contributing to the molecule's size, flexibility, and transport characteristics. Its small side chain allows glutathione to maintain a compact form that can diffuse through the cytosol and enter specific compartments where it is needed. This mobility is essential because reactive intermediates are generated in multiple locations, and the buffering system must be able to reach those sites without delay. Glycine does not carry the reactive or stabilizing properties of the other residues, but its presence ensures that the molecule can function within the spatial constraints of the cell. It allows glutathione to act as a distributed system rather than a fixed component tied to a single location.

The combination of these three residues produces a molecule that is both stable and reactive, capable of existing at high concentrations while remaining chemically active. The gamma-glutamyl bond preserves the molecule, the cysteine thiol enables interaction with reactive species, and the glycine residue supports movement and accessibility. This architecture allows glutathione to operate as a continuous buffer, absorbing reactive load as it is generated and returning to its reduced state through enzymatic recycling. The molecule does not act once and disappear. It cycles, maintaining conditions that allow other processes to proceed without disruption.

This structural design also determines how glutathione integrates into larger systems. Its stability allows it to accumulate within compartments such as the cytosol and mitochondria, where it supports localized redox balance. Its reactivity allows it to participate in detoxification by forming conjugates with electrophilic compounds, rendering them transportable and removable. Its mobility allows it to link these functions across different regions of the cell, ensuring that no single area becomes isolated from the buffering system. Each aspect of its structure contributes to a role that extends beyond a single reaction or pathway.

Understanding glutathione at this level removes the tendency to describe it as a general antioxidant and instead frames it as a molecule engineered for continuous participation in cellular stability. Its architecture is not a minimal arrangement of amino acids but a configuration that supports persistence, controlled reactivity, and system-wide distribution. These properties allow it to define the conditions under which cellular processes operate, ensuring that reactions are completed and that reactive intermediates do not accumulate within the system.

Glutamate → Protection and Stability

The glutamate residue defines how glutathione is preserved inside the cell and sets the conditions that allow it to function as a standing buffer rather than a transient peptide. Its placement at the front of the molecule creates a gamma-glutamyl linkage that deviates from the standard peptide bond used in most proteins. This difference is structural, not cosmetic. Cellular peptidases are built to recognize and cleave alpha-linked peptides, and they do so efficiently to recycle amino acids. The gamma linkage in glutathione is not recognized by these enzymes, which prevents rapid degradation and allows the molecule to persist at high intracellular concentrations. This resistance to breakdown is what gives glutathione its baseline presence across tissues, maintaining a continuous pool that can respond immediately to reactive load without waiting for new synthesis.

Protection, in this context, is not an active shielding mechanism but a consequence of maintained availability. Because glutathione is not constantly being degraded, the cell can hold a large reservoir of the molecule in its reduced form. This reservoir defines the buffering capacity of the system. When reactive intermediates are generated, they are met by an existing pool that can absorb them without delay. If glutathione were rapidly degraded like other small peptides, its levels would fluctuate with synthesis rates, and the system would be forced to operate with intermittent gaps in protection. The glutamate residue prevents this by stabilizing the molecule against enzymatic breakdown, ensuring that the buffering system is always present rather than conditionally assembled.

This stability also supports compartmental organization. Different regions of the cell maintain their own glutathione pools, and these pools must remain intact under varying conditions of stress and metabolic activity. The resistance to degradation allows glutathione to accumulate within these compartments and remain available even when local conditions shift. In the mitochondria, where reactive species are generated continuously, this persistence is critical. The system cannot rely on constant synthesis to match demand. It requires a pre-existing concentration that can absorb fluctuations in reactive output. The structural role of glutamate makes this possible by preventing loss of the molecule through routine peptide turnover.

The gamma-glutamyl structure also influences how glutathione interacts with transport and recycling systems. Its stability allows it to circulate within intracellular spaces and participate in repeated cycles of oxidation and reduction without being broken down between cycles. This continuity supports the enzymatic systems that regenerate reduced glutathione from its oxidized form, maintaining a consistent ratio that defines the redox environment. The molecule remains intact as it moves through these cycles, preserving its functional capacity over time.

Glutamate, therefore, does not contribute to reactivity in the same way as cysteine, but it determines whether that reactivity can be sustained within the system. By protecting the molecule from degradation, it ensures that glutathione exists as a persistent structural component of cellular chemistry. This persistence allows the cell to maintain a stable redox environment under continuous metabolic activity, preventing gaps in buffering capacity and supporting the completion of reactions as they occur.

Cysteine → Reactive Sulfur Core

The cysteine residue defines what glutathione actually does. Its thiol group carries a sulfur atom that holds electrons in a state that can be transferred, accepted, and rebalanced without collapsing the molecule.

This is not a passive feature. It is the active site where reactive intermediates are intercepted and converted into controlled forms. Oxygen-derived species, electrophiles generated during detoxification, and oxidized protein residues all converge on this sulfur center because it can engage them directly. The interaction is immediate and local. When a reactive species encounters glutathione, the cysteine thiol donates an electron and shifts into an oxidized state, forming a disulfide linkage with another glutathione molecule. This conversion captures the reactive load and prevents it from propagating into surrounding structures.

The behavior of this sulfur group determines how effectively the cell can contain reactivity as it is generated. In its reduced form, the thiol remains available to engage new intermediates. In its oxidized form, it represents stored oxidative load that must be resolved through enzymatic reduction. This creates a continuous cycle where glutathione absorbs reactive species and is then restored to its functional state by glutathione reductase using NADPH as the electron source. The cysteine residue is the point of exchange in this cycle. Without it, the molecule would retain stability from glutamate and mobility from glycine, but it would have no capacity to interact with reactive chemistry. The entire function of glutathione as a redox buffer depends on this sulfur center.

This reactivity is controlled rather than indiscriminate. The thiol group interacts with specific classes of molecules based on their electron configuration and chemical accessibility. It does not randomly neutralize everything it encounters. Instead, it participates in defined reactions that integrate into existing pathways. In detoxification, the cysteine thiol forms conjugates with electrophilic compounds, creating stable products that can be transported out of the cell. In protein regulation, it can reduce oxidized thiol groups on enzymes, restoring their active configuration. These interactions are selective and reversible, allowing the system to maintain flexibility while preventing accumulation of damage.

The sulfur atom also influences the broader redox environment by interacting with protein thiol networks. Many proteins contain cysteine residues that act as sensors and switches, changing configuration based on their oxidation state. Glutathione participates in maintaining these residues in a reduced state or in facilitating controlled oxidation when signaling requires it. This extends its influence beyond direct neutralization of reactive species into the regulation of enzyme activity and signaling pathways. The cysteine core allows glutathione to interface with these systems at the level where structural changes occur.

The efficiency of this system depends on maintaining the cysteine thiol in its reduced form. When the rate of oxidation exceeds the rate of recycling, the pool of reduced glutathione declines and the system loses its ability to intercept new reactive intermediates. This is where the function of the cysteine residue reveals its limits. It can absorb reactive load, but it must be continuously restored to remain effective. The presence of the sulfur core is necessary, but it is not sufficient on its own. It requires a surrounding system that supplies electrons for reduction and substrates for regeneration.

Cysteine, therefore, is not just one component of the molecule. It is the operational center that converts glutathione from a stable peptide into an active participant in cellular chemistry. Its sulfur group provides the interface between metabolic activity and structural preservation, allowing the cell to process reactive intermediates without allowing them to disrupt the system.

Glycine → Mobility and Distribution

Glycine determines how glutathione moves through the cell and how widely its buffering capacity can be applied. The residue itself does not carry a reactive side chain or provide structural protection in the way glutamate does, but its size and neutrality shape the physical behavior of the molecule. Glycine has no side chain beyond a hydrogen atom, which minimizes steric hindrance and allows the tripeptide to remain compact and flexible. This compact form reduces resistance as glutathione diffuses through the cytosol and enters transport systems that move it between compartments. The result is a molecule that can reach sites of reactive generation quickly rather than remaining localized to a single region.

This mobility is necessary because reactive intermediates are not produced in one place. Mitochondria generate them during electron transport, detoxification pathways produce them in the cytosol and endoplasmic reticulum, and membrane-associated processes create localized oxidative pressure at lipid interfaces. A buffering system that cannot distribute across these regions would leave gaps where reactive species could accumulate. Glycine enables glutathione to function as a distributed network rather than a fixed reservoir. It allows the molecule to be present wherever reactive load emerges, maintaining continuity of protection across spatially separated processes.

Transport mechanisms rely on this structural simplicity. Glutathione must pass through intracellular environments and, in some cases, across membranes via specific carriers. A larger or more structurally complex residue in place of glycine would alter the conformation of the molecule and reduce its ability to move efficiently through these systems. The glycine residue keeps the molecule within a size and shape range that supports rapid exchange between compartments. This is particularly important for maintaining mitochondrial glutathione pools, which depend on import from the cytosol. Efficient transport ensures that compartments with high reactive output can sustain their buffering capacity without delay.

Distribution also affects how glutathione participates in recycling and conjugation pathways. After oxidation or conjugation reactions, the molecule must either be restored to its reduced form or transported for further processing. Glycine supports this turnover by allowing glutathione to move between enzymes and pathways without structural constraints. The molecule does not become trapped in one functional state or location. It remains accessible to the systems that regenerate it or utilize it for detoxification, maintaining continuity of function across cycles.

The contribution of glycine becomes more apparent when considering what would happen in its absence. A less mobile molecule would create localized pools of buffering capacity, leaving other regions exposed to reactive accumulation. Even if total cellular glutathione levels were sufficient, uneven distribution would allow compartment-specific failure to occur. Glycine prevents this by ensuring that the molecule can diffuse, be transported, and be reused across the entire intracellular space. It supports a uniform redox environment rather than isolated pockets of stability.

Glycine does not directly engage reactive species, but it determines whether the molecule that does can be positioned where it is needed. Its role is spatial rather than chemical, enabling glutathione to operate as a system-wide component rather than a localized factor. Through this contribution, the tripeptide maintains continuous coverage across the cell, allowing reactive intermediates to be intercepted regardless of where they are generated.

Structure Determines Function

The behavior of glutathione is set by how its three residues are arranged, not by the presence of those residues alone. Glutamate establishes persistence through a gamma linkage that resists routine peptide cleavage, cysteine provides the sulfur center that can accept and donate electrons, and glycine maintains a compact geometry that allows the molecule to move between compartments and engage multiple systems without restriction. These elements do not act independently. Their combination creates a molecule that can exist at high concentration, remain chemically active, and cycle continuously between states without being consumed. This configuration defines what glutathione can do inside the cell and what it cannot.

Function emerges from how this structure interacts with the cellular environment. The protected backbone allows glutathione to remain intact long enough to act as a standing reservoir. The cysteine thiol engages reactive intermediates as they are formed, converting unstable species into controlled states. The small size permits rapid diffusion and transport, allowing the molecule to reach regions where reactive load is highest. When these features operate together, glutathione maintains a distributed buffering system that stabilizes reactions across compartments. The molecule does not target a single pathway. It sets the conditions under which many pathways can proceed without generating uncontrolled byproducts.

Altering any part of this structure changes system behavior. If the gamma-glutamyl linkage is removed, the molecule becomes susceptible to degradation, reducing its intracellular concentration and collapsing buffering capacity. If the cysteine thiol is modified or unavailable, the molecule loses its ability to interact with reactive species, leaving intermediates uncontained. If the overall size or conformation is changed, mobility decreases and distribution becomes uneven, allowing localized accumulation of reactive load. Each structural component contributes to a specific requirement, and the loss of any one of them disrupts the entire function.

This relationship between structure and function extends beyond glutathione itself. The molecule interacts with enzymes, membranes, and transport systems that recognize its specific configuration. Glutathione peroxidase relies on the availability of the reduced thiol to convert peroxides into less reactive forms. Glutathione reductase restores the oxidized molecule using NADPH, preserving the cycle. Transporters move glutathione into mitochondria and across membranes based on its size and charge distribution. These interactions are not interchangeable. They depend on the molecule maintaining its defined structure, which allows it to integrate into multiple systems simultaneously.

The outcome of this architecture is a molecule that operates continuously rather than episodically. It absorbs reactive load, is restored, and repeats the cycle without being depleted under normal conditions. This allows the cell to maintain a stable internal environment even as metabolic activity generates constant chemical flux. The structure does not simply enable function. It constrains it into a form that supports persistence, reversibility, and system-wide distribution. Without this configuration, glutathione would not be able to maintain the conditions required for cellular processes to complete without disruption.

Chapter 4

The Gamma-Glutamyl Bond

The defining structural feature of glutathione is the bond that connects glutamate to cysteine. This connection does not follow the standard pattern used in most peptides. Instead of linking through the typical position on the glutamate backbone, it forms through a different site, creating what is known as a gamma-glutamyl bond. This shift in connection point changes how the molecule is recognized by enzymes, how long it persists inside the cell, and how it participates in metabolic cycles. The bond is not a minor variation. It determines whether glutathione behaves like a transient peptide or a stable component of cellular architecture.

Most peptides in the body are built using a uniform linkage that enzymes can easily identify and break apart. This allows the cell to recycle amino acids efficiently and prevents unnecessary accumulation of small peptide fragments. Glutathione avoids this system by using a bond that falls outside the recognition pattern of these enzymes. As a result, it is not rapidly degraded and can maintain high intracellular concentrations. This persistence is required for its role as a redox buffer. The cell does not have to continuously rebuild glutathione to maintain function. Instead, it holds a standing pool that is ready to absorb reactive load as it is generated.

The gamma-glutamyl bond also allows glutathione to participate in a controlled cycle rather than a one-directional pathway. When the cysteine residue interacts with reactive species, the molecule becomes oxidized but remains intact. It is then restored to its reduced form through enzymatic action without being broken down into its individual amino acids. The bond ensures that glutathione can move through repeated cycles of oxidation and reduction without structural loss. This continuous reuse is what allows it to function as a system-level stabilizer rather than a consumable substrate.

This structural feature extends into the gamma-glutamyl cycle, a broader system that manages the movement and utilization of glutathione and related amino acids. The bond allows glutathione to interact with enzymes that transfer the gamma-glutamyl group to other molecules, facilitating transport and recycling processes. These interactions are specific to the bond's configuration. Without it, the molecule would not integrate into this cycle, and the system that maintains glutathione availability across tissues would not function in the same way.

The resistance to degradation also supports compartmental stability. Glutathione pools within the cytosol and mitochondria must remain intact under varying conditions of stress and metabolic activity. If the molecule were susceptible to rapid breakdown, these pools would fluctuate and leave periods where buffering capacity is reduced. The gamma-glutamyl bond prevents this by preserving the molecule even when demand is high, allowing the system to rely on a consistent baseline rather than intermittent synthesis.

The bond's position also influences how glutathione interacts with transport systems. Its structure allows it to be recognized by specific carriers that move it across membranes and into compartments where it is needed. This contributes to the distribution of glutathione throughout the cell and ensures that areas with high reactive output, such as the mitochondria, can maintain their own buffering capacity. The molecule's stability during transport prevents loss of function as it moves between locations.

Understanding the gamma-glutamyl bond shifts the view of glutathione from a simple tripeptide to a molecule engineered for persistence and reuse. The bond protects it from degradation, supports continuous cycling, and integrates it into systems that manage its distribution and availability. These properties allow glutathione to maintain a stable redox environment across the cell, ensuring that reactive intermediates are contained and that cellular processes can proceed without accumulating damage.

In Laymen's Terms

The most important feature of glutathione is how its first two pieces are connected. While this might seem like a small detail, it completely changes how the molecule behaves inside the body. Most small chains in the body are built in a standard way, and because of that, the body can easily break them apart and recycle them. Glutathione is different. The first connection, between glutamate and cysteine, is built in an unusual way that the body does not easily recognize or break down.

You can think of this like building something with a different type of connector that standard tools cannot undo. Because of this, glutathione stays intact much longer than most similar molecules. This matters because the body needs glutathione to always be present. It is not something that gets used once and thrown away. It needs to be available at all times to handle stress inside the cell. This special connection allows the body to keep a steady supply instead of constantly rebuilding it from scratch.

This same feature also allows glutathione to be reused over and over again. When it handles stress, it temporarily changes form, but it does not fall apart. The body can restore it back to its original state and use it again. Without this connection, glutathione would break down after each use, and the body would struggle to keep up with demand.

There is also a system in the body that helps move and recycle glutathione and its parts. This system depends on that unique connection. It allows glutathione to interact with other processes that help transport it where it is needed and keep it functioning properly. Without this structure, that system would not work the same way, and glutathione would not be as effective.

This connection also helps glutathione stay stable in different parts of the cell. Some areas of the cell produce more stress than others, especially the parts responsible for making energy. Those areas need a constant supply of glutathione. Because it does not break down easily, it can stay available in those places even when demand is high.

In simple terms, this special connection makes glutathione durable, reusable, and always available. Without it, the molecule would behave like any other small chain in the body, breaking down quickly and losing its ability to protect the cell over time.

Resistance to Degradation

Glutathione remains available inside the cell because its structure prevents it from being broken down by the same mechanisms that recycle most small peptides. Cellular enzymes are designed to recognize and cleave standard peptide bonds, allowing amino acids to be reused as needed. The gamma-glutamyl linkage at the front of glutathione falls outside that recognition pattern. As a result, the molecule is not rapidly dismantled during normal turnover. This resistance is not a passive feature. It defines how much glutathione can accumulate and how reliably it can be maintained under changing conditions.

A stable pool changes how the system behaves. When glutathione is preserved, the cell can hold a large amount of it in its reduced form, creating a standing buffer that absorbs reactive intermediates as they are generated. There is no delay between the production of reactive species and their containment because the buffering capacity is already in place. If glutathione were degraded at the same rate as other peptides, its concentration would fluctuate with synthesis, and the system would operate with intermittent gaps in protection. Those gaps would allow reactive intermediates to interact with proteins and membranes before being neutralized, increasing the likelihood of structural damage.

This resistance also reduces the metabolic cost of maintaining redox balance. Continuous synthesis would require a constant supply of amino acids and enzymatic activity, diverting resources from other processes. By preserving the molecule, the cell shifts from a model of constant replacement to one of reuse. Glutathione can cycle between reduced and oxidized forms without being broken down, allowing the same molecule to participate in repeated reactions. The system maintains function through recycling rather than consumption, which stabilizes both resource use and performance.

Compartmental stability depends on this persistence. Mitochondria, in particular, require a consistent glutathione pool to manage the reactive species generated during electron transport. These compartments cannot rely on rapid synthesis to meet immediate demand. They require a pre-existing concentration that remains intact even as conditions fluctuate. Resistance to degradation ensures that these localized pools do not collapse under stress, allowing each compartment to maintain its own buffering capacity.

The preserved structure also supports integration with transport and recycling systems. Because glutathione remains intact, it can move between compartments and interact with enzymes that restore it to its reduced state. The molecule does not need to be rebuilt after each reaction. It remains part of a continuous cycle, maintaining the redox environment across the cell without interruption.

Resistance to degradation therefore determines whether glutathione functions as a transient molecule or as a persistent component of cellular architecture. By avoiding rapid breakdown, it allows the cell to maintain a stable buffering system that operates continuously, ensuring that reactive intermediates are contained as they are formed and that cellular processes proceed without accumulating damage.Preservation vs consumption

Integration with Amino Acid Metabolism

Glutathione does not exist outside of amino acid metabolism. It is built from the same substrate pool that supports protein synthesis, energy production, and neurotransmitter formation, and it competes for those inputs in real time. The cell does not allocate amino acids in isolation. It distributes them based on demand across multiple systems, which means glutathione synthesis is directly tied to overall metabolic state. When amino acid availability is sufficient, the system can maintain both structural protein turnover and redox buffering. When availability is constrained, tradeoffs emerge, and glutathione production becomes limited by the same factors that restrict broader metabolic function.

Cysteine defines the primary bottleneck in this process. It is not abundant in free form within the cell and must either be obtained from the diet or generated through conversion pathways that depend on other nutrients. When cysteine supply is limited, glutathione synthesis slows regardless of how much glutamate and glycine are present. This creates a direct link between sulfur amino acid metabolism and redox capacity. The cell cannot increase glutathione production beyond what cysteine availability allows, which means any disruption in sulfur handling immediately reduces buffering capacity.

Glycine contributes to this integration through its role in multiple pathways that compete for its use. It participates in protein synthesis, collagen formation, and one-carbon metabolism, where it supports methylation reactions. When demand in these areas increases, less glycine is available for glutathione production. This does not eliminate synthesis but reduces the rate at which the system can maintain or restore its pool. The distribution of glycine therefore influences how quickly glutathione can respond to increased reactive load.

Glutamate is more readily available, but its role connects glutathione to central metabolic flux. It is involved in nitrogen handling and links amino acid metabolism to the tricarboxylic acid cycle through transamination reactions. This places glutathione synthesis within the broader context of energy metabolism and nitrogen balance. Changes in glutamate availability or utilization can shift how resources are allocated between energy production and redox buffering, especially under conditions of stress where both systems are under increased demand.

The integration extends beyond synthesis into recycling and transport. When glutathione is broken down or exported, its amino acid components re-enter the metabolic pool and can be reused or redirected. The gamma-glutamyl cycle facilitates this exchange, allowing the cell to recover amino acids while maintaining overall glutathione function. This creates a feedback system where glutathione metabolism and amino acid availability influence each other continuously rather than operating as separate processes.

Because glutathione depends on the same inputs as other essential functions, its levels reflect the state of the entire metabolic network. Adequate amino acid intake supports sustained synthesis and stable redox conditions. Deficiency or imbalance reduces production and shifts the system toward reliance on existing stores and recycling. When demand exceeds both synthesis and recycling capacity, glutathione levels decline and the cell loses its ability to fully resolve reactive intermediates.

This relationship places glutathione at the intersection of structural metabolism and chemical stability. It is not produced independently of the system but emerges from it, drawing from the same resources that support growth, repair, and energy generation. Its availability therefore signals whether the cell has sufficient substrate and capacity to maintain internal order under ongoing metabolic activity.

Chapter 5

Redox Chemistry and Controlled Reactivity

Redox chemistry describes the movement of electrons through the cell, but in a living system this movement cannot be left unregulated. Every transfer of electrons creates transitional states where molecules are temporarily unstable and capable of reacting with nearby structures. These intermediates are necessary for metabolism, yet they carry the potential to disrupt proteins, lipids, and nucleic acids if they persist. The cell must therefore manage not only where electrons go, but how long reactive states are allowed to exist. Controlled reactivity is the mechanism that keeps these processes contained, allowing reactions to proceed without spreading instability across the system.

Glutathione operates at the center of this control because it can accept and donate electrons in a reversible and repeatable manner. Its cysteine thiol serves as the exchange point where reactive species are intercepted and converted into a stable form. When a reactive molecule encounters glutathione, the thiol donates an electron and becomes oxidized, forming a disulfide bond. This captures the reactive intermediate and prevents it from interacting with other cellular components. The oxidized form is not the end state. It is a temporary storage of reactive load that can be reversed through enzymatic reduction. This reversibility allows the system to absorb fluctuations in reactive production without losing capacity over time.

The distinction between controlled and uncontrolled reactivity lies in timing and containment. In a controlled system, reactive intermediates are generated and resolved within tightly defined boundaries. They exist long enough to complete their role in a reaction and are then neutralized or incorporated into stable products. In an uncontrolled system, these intermediates persist beyond their intended context, interacting with unintended targets and initiating secondary reactions. This leads to a cascade where one unresolved intermediate produces others, amplifying the disruption. The difference is not the presence of reactive species but whether the system can terminate their activity at the correct point.

Enzymatic systems extend this control by directing how reactive intermediates are processed. Glutathione peroxidase uses reduced glutathione to convert peroxides into less reactive compounds, preventing them from initiating lipid peroxidation or protein oxidation. Glutathione reductase restores oxidized glutathione using NADPH, maintaining the pool of reduced molecules required for continued buffering. These enzymes do not act independently. Their activity depends on the availability of glutathione and reducing equivalents, linking redox control to broader metabolic systems. When any part of this network is constrained, the ability to maintain controlled reactivity declines.

Compartmentalization adds another layer of regulation. Different regions of the cell operate under different redox conditions, reflecting their specific functions. The mitochondria generate a continuous flow of reactive species as part of energy production and require a dedicated system to contain them. The cytosol maintains a broader buffering environment that stabilizes reactions across multiple pathways. These compartments are not isolated. Changes in one region can influence others through shared metabolites and signaling pathways. Controlled reactivity depends on maintaining appropriate conditions within each compartment while allowing coordination across the system.

The concept of controlled reactivity also explains how redox chemistry participates in signaling rather than only in damage. Certain proteins respond to changes in redox state by altering their configuration, which can activate or deactivate specific pathways. These changes must be reversible and limited in scope to function as signals rather than disruptions. Glutathione contributes to this by maintaining a baseline redox environment and by restoring proteins to their reduced state after signaling events. Without this restoration, signaling pathways would remain locked in an activated or deactivated state, losing their ability to respond dynamically.

When redox control is intact, the cell can operate under continuous chemical flux without accumulating damage. Reactions proceed, intermediates are resolved, and the system returns to baseline conditions after each cycle. When control is lost, the same reactions produce a growing pool of unresolved intermediates that alter structure and function across the cell. The transition from stability to instability is defined by the system's ability to manage electron flow and terminate reactive states. Glutathione does not eliminate reactivity. It shapes it, ensuring that the chemical processes required for life remain contained within boundaries that preserve cellular integrity.

Electron Donation and Recovery

Glutathione functions by taking on reactive load and then returning to a usable state, and both halves of that cycle have to remain intact for the system to work. The donation phase begins at the cysteine thiol, where electrons are held in a form that can be transferred to reactive intermediates as they appear. When a peroxide, free radical, or electrophilic compound enters the intracellular environment, glutathione meets it directly and donates an electron, converting that unstable species into a less reactive form. This transfer stabilizes the intermediate and prevents it from interacting with proteins, lipids, or DNA. At the same time, glutathione itself is altered. Two molecules link together through a disulfide bond, forming the oxidized state. The reactive load has not disappeared. It has been captured and stored in a controlled configuration.

That storage state only preserves system stability if it can be reversed. Recovery depends on glutathione reductase and a continuous supply of reducing equivalents in the form of NADPH. The enzyme breaks the disulfide bond and returns glutathione to its reduced form, restoring the thiol group so it can participate in another cycle of electron donation. This is not an occasional repair step. It operates continuously, matching the rate at which glutathione is oxidized. The system maintains a balance where most of the pool remains in the reduced state, ensuring that reactive intermediates can be intercepted as they are generated.

The efficiency of this cycle determines how much reactive load the cell can manage without disruption. If donation proceeds faster than recovery, the pool shifts toward the oxidized form and the availability of reduced glutathione declines. As this shift progresses, new reactive intermediates encounter fewer available thiol groups and begin to persist in the intracellular environment. This marks the transition from controlled to uncontrolled reactivity. The system has not stopped functioning, but it has lost the ability to keep up with the rate of electron transfer required to maintain stability.

NADPH supply sets the upper limit for recovery. It is generated through metabolic pathways that also support biosynthesis and energy balance, linking redox control to broader cellular function. When NADPH production is sufficient, oxidized glutathione is rapidly reduced and the cycle continues without interruption. When it is limited, recovery slows and the oxidized pool accumulates. This creates a bottleneck where the system can still donate electrons but cannot restore its capacity quickly enough to handle ongoing demand.

Compartmental dynamics further influence this process. Mitochondria rely on localized glutathione pools to manage the reactive species generated during electron transport, and these pools depend on both import of reduced glutathione and local recycling. If recovery is impaired within this compartment, reactive intermediates begin to damage mitochondrial components, reducing energy output and increasing further reactive production. The imbalance between donation and recovery propagates through the system, affecting other compartments that depend on mitochondrial function.

The cycle of electron donation and recovery defines glutathione as a reusable system rather than a consumable molecule. It absorbs reactive load, stores it temporarily, and then returns to its active state to repeat the process. Stability depends on maintaining both sides of this cycle at matched rates. When donation and recovery remain balanced, reactive intermediates are contained and resolved. When they diverge, the system accumulates oxidative load and begins to lose control over the reactions it initiates.

Reversible Oxidation (GSH ↔ GSSG)

Glutathione operates through a controlled shift between two states, reduced glutathione and oxidized glutathione, and this transition defines how the cell handles reactive load. In its reduced form, glutathione carries an available thiol group on the cysteine residue, positioned to donate electrons to reactive intermediates. When that donation occurs, two glutathione molecules link together through a disulfide bond, forming the oxidized state. This conversion does not destroy the molecule. It captures the reactive burden in a stable configuration that can be reversed. The system uses this transition as a way to temporarily store oxidative load while preventing it from interacting with critical structures.

The ratio between these two forms determines the redox environment of the cell. A high proportion of reduced glutathione maintains conditions where proteins retain their functional structure, enzymes operate efficiently, and signaling pathways respond within defined limits. As the oxidized form accumulates, this balance shifts. Thiol groups on proteins begin to form disulfide bonds, altering their configuration and reducing activity. Membrane components become more susceptible to oxidative modification, and signaling systems that depend on redox-sensitive switches begin to deviate from their normal patterns. The change in ratio does not simply reflect stress. It actively drives changes in cellular behavior.

Reversibility depends on continuous reduction of oxidized glutathione back to its active form. Glutathione reductase carries out this process using NADPH as the electron source, breaking the disulfide bond and restoring two molecules of reduced glutathione. This step closes the loop, allowing the system to recycle its buffering capacity rather than depleting it. The efficiency of this reduction determines how quickly the cell can recover from oxidative events and return to baseline conditions. When reduction keeps pace with oxidation, the pool remains predominantly in the reduced state and the system maintains stability.

If oxidation outpaces reduction, the balance shifts toward the oxidized form and the availability of reduced glutathione declines. This creates a condition where new reactive intermediates encounter fewer available thiol groups and persist longer within the cell. The system begins to accumulate unresolved intermediates, and the redox environment moves away from a state that supports normal function. The shift is not binary. It progresses as the ratio changes, with increasing effects on enzyme activity, membrane integrity, and signaling behavior.

Compartmental differences add complexity to this transition. The cytosol, mitochondria, and other regions maintain their own glutathione pools and can experience different ratios at the same time. A localized increase in oxidized glutathione within mitochondria can impair energy production even if the overall cellular ratio appears stable. These compartment-specific shifts can propagate through the system, linking local imbalance to broader dysfunction.

The reversible nature of the GSH to GSSG transition allows the cell to absorb and release oxidative load without permanent loss of capacity. It functions as a dynamic buffer that adjusts to changes in demand while maintaining the conditions required for cellular processes to proceed. Stability depends on keeping this cycle intact and maintaining a ratio that supports continuous function. When that balance is preserved, reactive intermediates are contained and resolved. When it is disrupted, the same intermediates begin to accumulate and alter the system from within.

Precision vs Indiscriminate Antioxidant Behavior

Glutathione does not function as a broad, uncontrolled scavenger that neutralizes everything it encounters. Its activity is directed by chemical compatibility, enzymatic context, and cellular location, which together determine when and where it engages reactive intermediates. The cysteine thiol does not randomly donate electrons. It interacts with specific classes of molecules that present the correct electronic structure and accessibility. Many of these interactions are mediated or accelerated by enzymes such as glutathione peroxidase and glutathione S-transferases, which guide the reaction toward defined outcomes. This creates a system where reactivity is applied with selectivity, ensuring that necessary signaling events and controlled oxidative processes are not disrupted.

Indiscriminate antioxidant behavior would collapse normal cellular function. Reactive species are not only byproducts of metabolism. They are also used in signaling pathways that regulate gene expression, immune activation, and adaptive responses to stress. These signals depend on transient, localized changes in redox state. If all reactive intermediates were neutralized immediately and without discrimination, these signaling mechanisms would fail. The cell would lose the ability to detect and respond to changes in its environment. Glutathione avoids this by operating within boundaries defined by concentration, location, and enzyme interaction. It allows controlled reactivity to occur while preventing that reactivity from spreading beyond its intended scope.

Enzymatic coupling is central to this precision. Glutathione peroxidase uses reduced glutathione to convert specific peroxides into less reactive compounds, targeting molecules that would otherwise initiate chain reactions such as lipid peroxidation. Glutathione S-transferases facilitate conjugation with electrophilic compounds, directing glutathione toward detoxification pathways. These enzymes create defined entry points where glutathione engages reactive intermediates under controlled conditions. Outside of these contexts, its activity is limited by diffusion, concentration gradients, and chemical compatibility, which prevents it from acting as a universal scavenger.

Spatial organization further refines this behavior. Glutathione concentrations differ between compartments, and its interactions are influenced by the local environment. In mitochondria, where reactive species are generated continuously, the system is tuned to intercept those intermediates before they damage membrane components. In the cytosol, the buffering capacity is broader but still regulated, maintaining conditions that support enzyme function without suppressing necessary signaling. This compartmental control ensures that glutathione acts where it is needed without interfering with processes that rely on transient oxidative states.

The distinction between precision and indiscriminate action becomes clear when examining how the system responds to increased demand. When reactive load rises within manageable limits, glutathione engages targeted pathways to contain and resolve intermediates. When the load exceeds capacity, reactive species begin to escape these controlled interactions and spread through the cell, initiating secondary reactions that are no longer regulated. The system does not become more active in a precise way. It becomes overwhelmed, and reactivity shifts from controlled to diffuse.

Glutathione's role is therefore not to eliminate reactivity but to shape it. It allows specific reactions to occur while preventing those reactions from extending beyond their intended boundaries. This selective engagement preserves both the functional use of reactive intermediates in signaling and the structural integrity of the cell. Precision defines the system's ability to maintain balance, ensuring that reactivity remains a tool rather than a source of uncontrolled damage.

PART III

CELLULAR ARCHITECTURE → SYSTEM PLACEMENT

Where glutathione operates and why position matters

Chapter 6

Intracellular Distribution

Glutathione does not function as a single uniform pool spread evenly throughout the cell. It is distributed across compartments, and each compartment maintains its own concentration, redox ratio, and functional role. This distribution determines how effectively reactive intermediates are contained and how different parts of the cell maintain stability under metabolic load. The system operates as a set of localized buffering environments rather than a single shared reservoir. Movement between these environments is regulated, and each compartment depends on its own balance between supply, consumption, and recovery.

The cytosol holds the largest portion of glutathione and sets the baseline redox environment for the cell. Most synthesis occurs here, drawing from available amino acids and using ATP-dependent steps to assemble the molecule. The cytosolic pool interacts with a wide range of enzymes and substrates, maintaining conditions that support protein function and metabolic reactions. Because of its volume and accessibility, it acts as the primary buffer that absorbs fluctuations in reactive load generated across multiple pathways. However, this pool cannot fully compensate for localized demands in other compartments where reactive species are produced at higher rates.

Mitochondria maintain a separate glutathione pool that is critical for controlling the reactive intermediates generated during electron transport. This pool is not synthesized locally. It is imported from the cytosol through specific transport systems that move glutathione across the mitochondrial membranes. Once inside, it must be maintained through local recycling because rapid replacement from the cytosol is limited. The mitochondrial environment produces a continuous flow of reactive species, and without a stable internal pool, these intermediates would interact with membrane lipids and respiratory complexes, impairing energy production and increasing further reactive output. The balance within this compartment determines whether energy generation proceeds efficiently or becomes a source of escalating instability.

The endoplasmic reticulum operates under a different redox condition, supporting processes that require controlled oxidation, such as protein folding and disulfide bond formation. Glutathione participates here by maintaining a balance that allows these reactions to occur without spreading oxidative stress beyond the intended context. The ratio of reduced to oxidized glutathione in this compartment differs from that of the cytosol, reflecting its specialized function. This illustrates that glutathione distribution is not only spatial but also functional, with each compartment tuned to its specific requirements.

The nucleus relies on glutathione to maintain the structural integrity of DNA and the function of regulatory proteins. Redox-sensitive transcription factors respond to changes in the local environment, and glutathione helps restore these proteins to their active configurations after signaling events. While the nuclear pool is influenced by the cytosolic environment, it must remain stable enough to protect genetic material from reactive intermediates that could alter its structure.

Transport between compartments is selective and controlled. Glutathione does not diffuse freely across membranes. Carrier systems and gradients determine how it moves, ensuring that compartments maintain distinct conditions rather than equilibrating into a single uniform state. This separation allows each region to operate within parameters suited to its function while still being connected to the broader system.

When intracellular distribution is intact, each compartment maintains the buffering capacity required for its specific processes, and reactive intermediates are contained within defined boundaries. When distribution is disrupted, imbalances emerge. A depleted mitochondrial pool can lead to increased reactive production that affects the cytosol, while shifts in the endoplasmic reticulum can interfere with protein processing and signaling. These localized failures propagate through the system because compartments are interdependent.

Glutathione distribution therefore defines how the cell organizes its defense against reactive load. It is not the total amount alone that determines stability, but how that amount is partitioned, maintained, and coordinated across compartments. Each pool contributes to a network that contains reactivity at its source and preserves the structural and functional integrity of the cell.

Cytosol, Mitochondria, Nucleus, Membranes

Glutathione operates as a distributed system across the cell, and each location imposes different demands on how it is used, maintained, and recycled. The cytosol establishes the baseline environment. It contains the largest pool and serves as the primary site of synthesis, where glutathione is assembled from glutamate, cysteine, and glycine using ATP-dependent steps. This pool supports a wide range of enzymatic reactions and maintains protein thiols in a reduced state so that enzymes retain their functional shape. Because most metabolic pathways interface with the cytosol at some point, this compartment absorbs a constant background level of reactive intermediates. Its role is broad stabilization rather than targeted defense, maintaining conditions where reactions proceed without accumulating structural damage.

Mitochondria operate under a different constraint. Electron transport continuously generates reactive intermediates as electrons move through respiratory complexes. These intermediates form at the inner membrane, directly adjacent to lipid structures that are vulnerable to oxidation. The mitochondrial glutathione pool must therefore remain tightly maintained to intercept these species before they initiate chain reactions in membrane lipids. This pool is imported from the cytosol and then sustained through local recycling. When mitochondrial glutathione is sufficient, reactive intermediates are contained at their point of origin and energy production proceeds without disruption. When it declines, reactive species begin to alter membrane integrity and impair the function of respiratory complexes, reducing ATP output and increasing further reactive production in a self-amplifying cycle.

The nucleus depends on a stable redox environment to preserve DNA structure and regulate transcriptional activity. Reactive intermediates that reach this compartment can alter nucleotide bases or disrupt proteins that control gene expression. Glutathione maintains nuclear proteins in a reduced state, allowing transcription factors to bind and release DNA in a controlled manner. It also participates in restoring these proteins after redox-sensitive signaling events. The nuclear pool is influenced by the cytosolic environment but must remain sufficiently buffered to prevent transient changes in redox state from producing lasting alterations in genetic regulation.

Membranes introduce a different type of problem. Reactive intermediates interacting with lipids initiate chain reactions that propagate across the membrane surface, altering its structure and fluidity. Glutathione does not embed within the lipid bilayer, but it operates at the interface, working with enzymes that terminate these chain reactions before they spread. In mitochondria and other organelles, this interface becomes critical because membrane integrity determines the function of embedded proteins, including transporters and respiratory complexes. When glutathione-dependent systems contain these reactions early, membrane structure is preserved. When they fail, lipid peroxidation spreads and disrupts both barrier function and signaling.

These compartments do not function independently. The cytosolic pool supplies glutathione to mitochondria, influences nuclear conditions, and supports enzyme systems that protect membranes. A deficit in one region increases demand in others, shifting the overall balance of the system. The distribution of glutathione therefore defines how the cell allocates its buffering capacity across different structural and functional demands. Stability depends on maintaining each compartment within its required range while allowing coordinated exchange between them.

Compartment-Specific Demands

Each compartment of the cell imposes its own pattern of reactive load, and glutathione is shaped around those differences rather than applied uniformly. The cytosol carries a continuous, moderate demand driven by metabolic throughput. Glycolysis, amino acid turnover, and detoxification pathways all generate intermediates that require containment, but they do so across a wide volume with relatively diffuse intensity. The cytosolic glutathione pool is therefore sized for breadth. It maintains a high concentration of reduced molecules to stabilize protein structure, sustain enzyme activity, and absorb fluctuations that arise as multiple pathways intersect. Its demand is defined by constant exposure rather than acute spikes.

Mitochondria operate under concentrated, high-frequency demand. Reactive intermediates are generated directly at the inner membrane as electrons move through the respiratory chain, and these intermediates form in close proximity to lipid structures that can propagate chain reactions if left unresolved. The mitochondrial glutathione pool must act immediately and locally. Delay is not tolerated because diffusion allows these intermediates to interact with membrane lipids and protein complexes within the same space where they are generated. This creates a requirement for rapid cycling between reduced and oxidized forms, supported by local recovery systems. The demand is not only higher in intensity but also more tightly constrained in time and location.

The nucleus experiences a different type of requirement, defined less by volume of reactive production and more by sensitivity to disruption. DNA and regulatory proteins respond to changes in redox state, and even small deviations can alter transcriptional behavior. The nuclear glutathione pool must maintain a narrow range that preserves protein configuration while still allowing controlled redox signaling to occur. Excessive oxidation shifts transcription factors into inactive or altered states, while excessive reduction can suppress signaling events that depend on transient oxidative changes. The demand here is precision, maintaining a stable environment that supports regulated change without drift.

Membranes introduce a propagation problem. Reactive intermediates that reach lipid structures can initiate chain reactions that spread laterally across the bilayer, amplifying the initial event. The demand at membrane interfaces is therefore defined by containment speed. Glutathione-dependent systems must intercept and terminate these reactions at their earliest stage, preventing propagation rather than managing widespread damage after it occurs. This requires coordination with enzymes that operate at the membrane boundary, where lipid and aqueous environments meet. The effectiveness of this control determines whether membranes retain their structure and function or begin to lose integrity under sustained reactive pressure.

These demands are not static. They shift with changes in metabolic activity, substrate availability, and external stressors. Increased energy production raises mitochondrial demand, while exposure to electrophilic compounds increases cytosolic and membrane-associated load. The system adjusts by redistributing glutathione and altering the rate of synthesis and recycling, but this adjustment is constrained by substrate availability and enzymatic capacity. When demand in one compartment rises beyond what can be locally managed, it begins to draw from the broader system, affecting the balance elsewhere.

Compartment-specific demands therefore define how glutathione is used, not just where it is located. Each region requires a different balance between concentration, turnover, and recovery speed, and the system maintains stability by meeting those requirements simultaneously. When this balance holds, reactive intermediates are contained within their point of origin and resolved without spreading. When it breaks, localized overload propagates outward, linking compartmental failure into a system-wide shift in redox control.

Chapter 7

Mitochondrial Protection

Mitochondria generate energy by moving electrons through a series of membrane-bound complexes, and this process produces reactive intermediates as a direct consequence of electron flow. These intermediates form at the inner mitochondrial membrane, in immediate proximity to lipids and protein complexes that are essential for maintaining the proton gradient and ATP synthesis. The system cannot eliminate this reactivity because it is inherent to energy production. It must contain it at the point of origin and resolve it before it spreads. Mitochondrial protection is therefore defined by how effectively the cell controls these intermediates within a confined space where both generation and vulnerability are concentrated.

Glutathione provides the primary buffering system within this compartment, but it is not synthesized inside the mitochondria. It is imported from the cytosol through carrier systems and then maintained locally through recycling. This creates a dependency on both supply and recovery. The imported pool must be sufficient to meet baseline demand, and the local reduction systems must restore oxidized glutathione at a rate that matches ongoing electron leakage. The balance between these processes determines whether the mitochondrial environment remains stable or begins to accumulate unresolved intermediates.

At the inner membrane, reactive species interact first with lipid components that define membrane structure and fluidity. If these interactions are not contained, they initiate chain reactions that alter the membrane's physical properties and disrupt the function of embedded protein complexes. Glutathione-dependent enzymes intercept these intermediates and convert them into less reactive forms before propagation occurs. This action preserves the integrity of the membrane and maintains the conditions required for efficient electron transport. When this containment is effective, energy production proceeds without structural compromise.

The relationship between reactive production and containment is dynamic. Increased metabolic demand raises electron flow and increases the rate at which reactive intermediates are generated. The mitochondrial glutathione system must scale with this demand by increasing the rate of oxidation and subsequent recovery. If recovery through glutathione reductase and NADPH supply keeps pace, the system maintains a stable redox environment. If it does not, oxidized glutathione accumulates and the availability of reduced molecules declines. This reduces the capacity to intercept new intermediates, allowing them to persist and interact with mitochondrial components.

As containment weakens, the effects extend beyond the membrane. Protein complexes involved in electron transport begin to lose efficiency, increasing electron leakage and further reactive production. This creates a feedback loop where reduced energy output and increased reactive generation reinforce each other. The system shifts from controlled reactivity to self-amplifying instability, where each cycle of electron transport produces more disruption than the last.

Mitochondrial protection also influences signaling pathways that extend beyond the organelle. Changes in mitochondrial redox state can alter the release of signaling molecules and affect nuclear responses that regulate metabolism and stress adaptation. When glutathione maintains control within the mitochondria, these signals remain within functional ranges. When control is lost, signaling becomes distorted, linking local instability to broader cellular changes.

The effectiveness of mitochondrial protection is determined by the capacity to maintain a stable glutathione pool within this compartment and to match recovery with ongoing demand. It is not defined by eliminating reactive species but by containing them within boundaries that preserve membrane structure, protein function, and energy production. When this balance is maintained, mitochondria operate as stable energy systems. When it is disrupted, they become a source of escalating reactive load that propagates through the cell.

Electron Transport and ROS Containment

Electron transport is built around the controlled movement of electrons through a series of membrane-bound complexes, but this movement is never perfectly contained. A small fraction of electrons escape before reaching their final acceptor and interact with oxygen to form reactive species. This occurs primarily at specific points along the chain where electron density builds and transfer becomes less efficient. These escape events are not rare anomalies. They are a continuous byproduct of energy production, and their rate increases as electron flow rises or becomes imbalanced. The system must therefore operate with the expectation that reactive species will be generated and must be neutralized immediately within the same space.

These reactive intermediates form directly adjacent to the inner mitochondrial membrane, where respiratory complexes and lipid structures are tightly packed. The proximity means there is no buffer zone between generation and potential damage. If a reactive species is not intercepted, it can initiate lipid oxidation or alter protein structure within the same region where it was produced. Containment depends on maintaining a high local concentration of reduced glutathione and the enzymes that use it. Glutathione peroxidase converts peroxides into less reactive molecules, preventing them from initiating chain reactions in membrane lipids. This reaction consumes reduced glutathione, shifting it into the oxidized form and transferring the reactive load into a controlled state.

The system only remains stable if recovery matches this rate of consumption. Glutathione reductase restores oxidized glutathione using NADPH, re-establishing the pool of reduced molecules required for continued containment. This creates a closed loop where electron leakage produces reactive species, glutathione captures and neutralizes them, and enzymatic systems restore glutathione to its active form. The efficiency of this loop determines whether reactive intermediates remain confined or begin to accumulate.

Imbalance begins when the rate of reactive generation exceeds the combined capacity of glutathione and its recovery systems. As reduced glutathione declines, newly formed reactive species encounter fewer available thiol groups and persist longer within the membrane environment. This increases the probability of lipid peroxidation, where a single reactive event initiates a chain reaction that spreads across the membrane. As membrane integrity declines, electron transport becomes less efficient, increasing electron leakage and further reactive production. The system shifts into a feedback loop where containment failure amplifies the source of the problem.

Containment is therefore not a static property but a dynamic equilibrium between generation and resolution. Electron transport establishes the baseline production of reactive species, while glutathione defines how effectively that production is controlled. When the balance holds, reactive intermediates are resolved at the point of origin and do not propagate. When it fails, the same processes that generate energy begin to destabilize the structures required to produce it.

Energy Production vs Self-Damage

Mitochondria operate under a constraint that cannot be removed. The same electron flow that drives ATP production also creates the conditions for structural damage. Electrons move through the respiratory chain to establish a proton gradient, and this gradient powers ATP synthase. At the same time, a fraction of those electrons escape and react with oxygen, forming intermediates that can alter lipids and proteins within the inner membrane. The system is therefore built on a tradeoff. Increasing energy output increases the rate of electron movement, and with it, the probability of electron escape. The cell does not choose between energy and damage. It manages the boundary where one begins to compromise the other.

Glutathione defines that boundary by containing the reactive intermediates as they form. When reduced glutathione is abundant and recovery is matched to demand, the system absorbs the byproducts of electron transport without allowing them to accumulate. Electron flow can increase to meet energy requirements, and reactive intermediates are neutralized within the same compartment. The membrane maintains its structure, and the protein complexes embedded within it continue to operate efficiently. In this state, energy production scales without crossing into self-damage because containment keeps pace with generation.

The transition begins when containment lags behind production. As reduced glutathione is consumed and not restored quickly enough, reactive intermediates persist longer within the membrane environment. These intermediates begin to interact with lipid chains, initiating reactions that spread across the bilayer and alter its physical properties. Membrane fluidity changes, protein complexes lose alignment, and electron transfer becomes less efficient. This inefficiency increases electron leakage, which produces more reactive intermediates. The system moves from a controlled state into a feedback loop where energy production itself becomes a source of increasing damage.

At this point, the relationship between output and stability reverses. Additional demand for ATP drives higher electron flow, but the system can no longer contain the resulting intermediates. Energy production becomes less efficient even as demand increases, and more of the electron flow is diverted into reactive pathways rather than productive work. The mitochondria continue to operate, but the cost of that operation rises in the form of structural degradation and reduced output per unit of substrate.

NADPH availability sets a hard limit on how long the system can sustain high output without crossing this threshold. Recovery of oxidized glutathione depends on a continuous supply of reducing equivalents, linking mitochondrial protection to cytosolic metabolism and nutrient availability. When NADPH supply is sufficient, the system can maintain high rates of electron transport while preserving membrane integrity. When it is constrained, the recovery process slows, and the system reaches the point where reactive generation outpaces containment.

Energy production and self-damage are therefore not separate processes. They are coupled through the mechanics of electron movement and the capacity of the cell to contain its byproducts. Glutathione does not eliminate the tradeoff. It extends the range over which energy can be produced without structural compromise. The position of that boundary determines whether mitochondria function as stable energy systems or shift into a state where the act of producing energy progressively undermines the structures required to sustain it.

Chapter 8

Membrane and Lipid Protection

Cell membranes are built from lipid structures that define boundaries, control permeability, and organize protein function, and these structures exist in a state that is both stable and vulnerable. The same properties that allow membranes to remain fluid and responsive also make them susceptible to reactive intermediates generated within the cell. Lipid chains, particularly those with multiple double bonds, can be altered through oxidation, initiating reactions that spread across the membrane surface. Protection is therefore not about preventing all interaction with reactive species but about stopping those interactions before they propagate into structural disruption.

Glutathione operates at the aqueous interface surrounding membranes rather than within the lipid bilayer itself. Its role is to intercept reactive intermediates that reach the membrane boundary and convert them into forms that do not initiate chain reactions. This process is mediated through enzyme systems that use glutathione as a reducing agent to neutralize peroxides and other reactive compounds before they interact with lipid chains. By removing these intermediates at the point of contact, the system prevents the first step in a sequence that would otherwise spread across the membrane.

Lipid peroxidation follows a predictable pattern once initiated. A reactive intermediate alters a lipid chain, creating a new reactive site that can interact with adjacent lipids. This produces a chain reaction where each event generates another, allowing the process to move laterally through the membrane. As this progresses, the physical properties of the membrane change. Fluidity is altered, permeability increases, and the arrangement of embedded proteins becomes less stable. Transport systems and signaling receptors depend on the integrity of this structure, and disruption at the lipid level translates directly into functional impairment.

Glutathione-dependent systems terminate these reactions early by reducing lipid peroxides and preventing the formation of new reactive sites. This requires both sufficient concentration of reduced glutathione and the activity of enzymes positioned at or near the membrane interface. The timing of this intervention determines whether the reaction is contained or allowed to propagate. Early containment preserves the original structure, while delayed intervention must address a spreading process that has already altered multiple lipid molecules.

Membrane composition influences how easily these reactions begin and how quickly they spread. Lipids with higher degrees of unsaturation provide more points where reactive intermediates can initiate changes. This increases the importance of maintaining a strong glutathione system in environments where such lipids are present. The balance between membrane composition and buffering capacity defines the system's resistance to propagation. When buffering capacity matches or exceeds the susceptibility of the membrane, structural integrity is maintained. When it does not, the membrane becomes a site where reactive processes expand rather than resolve.

The relationship between membranes and mitochondria reinforces this dynamic. The inner mitochondrial membrane contains a high density of lipid structures directly involved in energy production, and disruption in this region affects both structural integrity and metabolic output. Reactive intermediates generated during electron transport encounter these lipids immediately, making rapid containment essential. Failure in this context links membrane damage directly to impaired energy production, creating a combined structural and functional deficit.

Membrane protection therefore depends on positioning glutathione and its associated systems at the interface where reactive intermediates meet lipid structures. It is not a generalized antioxidant effect but a localized containment strategy that prevents small events from becoming self-propagating processes. When this system is intact, membranes maintain their structure and support the functions built upon them. When it fails, the same properties that allow membranes to function dynamically become pathways for the spread of damage across the cell.

Lipid Peroxidation Control

Lipid peroxidation begins when a reactive intermediate removes an electron from a lipid chain, creating a lipid radical that can react with oxygen and propagate across the membrane. This is not a single event. It is a sequence where each altered lipid becomes a new source of reactivity, allowing the process to spread laterally through the bilayer. The rate of propagation depends on how quickly these intermediate states are resolved. If they persist, the reaction amplifies. If they are intercepted early, the sequence terminates before it expands.

Glutathione controls this process at the stage where lipid peroxides form. These peroxides are unstable intermediates that can either be reduced to stable products or break down into new reactive species that continue the chain. Glutathione peroxidase uses reduced glutathione to convert lipid peroxides into non-propagating forms, removing the intermediate that drives further reactions. This intervention occurs at the membrane interface, where lipid and aqueous environments meet. The reaction consumes reduced glutathione and produces its oxidized form, transferring the reactive burden into a contained state that can be reversed through enzymatic recovery.

The effectiveness of this control depends on timing and availability. Early reduction of lipid peroxides stops the chain before multiple lipids are affected. Delayed reduction allows the reaction to spread, increasing the number of altered lipids and creating a broader area of instability. As more lipid radicals form, the system requires more glutathione to contain them, increasing the rate of consumption and placing greater demand on recovery systems. If recovery does not match this demand, reduced glutathione declines and the capacity to terminate new reactions decreases.

Membrane composition influences how easily this process begins and how aggressively it propagates. Lipids with multiple double bonds provide more sites where reactive intermediates can initiate peroxidation. This increases both the likelihood of initiation and the speed of propagation. In membranes with higher susceptibility, the requirement for rapid glutathione-dependent reduction becomes more critical. The system must operate with minimal delay to prevent localized events from expanding into widespread structural disruption.

As lipid peroxidation progresses, the physical properties of the membrane change. The bilayer becomes less ordered, permeability increases, and embedded proteins lose alignment with their surrounding lipid environment. Transport systems become less efficient, signaling pathways become distorted, and in mitochondria, the function of respiratory complexes is impaired. These changes feed back into the system by increasing reactive production and reducing the efficiency of containment, reinforcing the propagation process.

Control of lipid peroxidation therefore depends on maintaining a high local availability of reduced glutathione and the enzymatic capacity to use it at the point where intermediates form. The system does not prevent the initial interaction between reactive species and lipids. It prevents that interaction from becoming a chain reaction. When containment is immediate, membrane structure remains intact. When it is delayed or insufficient, the reaction spreads and converts a localized event into a system-level disruption.

Interaction with Vitamin E and Lipid Systems

Membrane protection is not carried out by a single molecule acting in isolation. It is a coordinated system where different components operate in distinct regions and pass reactive load between them in a controlled sequence. Vitamin E is positioned within the lipid bilayer itself, embedded among the fatty acid chains where lipid peroxidation begins. Glutathione remains in the aqueous phase outside the membrane, unable to enter the lipid core but able to influence what happens at its boundary. Their interaction is defined by location. Vitamin E intercepts lipid radicals inside the membrane, while glutathione supports the processes that restore and sustain that interception.

When a lipid radical forms, vitamin E donates an electron to stabilize it, converting the radical into a non-propagating lipid species. In doing so, vitamin E becomes oxidized and loses its ability to continue protecting the membrane unless it is restored. This is where the system extends beyond the lipid phase. Other molecules, supported by glutathione-dependent pathways, return vitamin E to its active state. Glutathione does not directly interact with vitamin E within the membrane, but it maintains the reducing environment required for this regeneration process to occur through intermediary systems. Without this support, oxidized vitamin E would accumulate and membrane protection would decline even if initial interception is effective.

This creates a layered defense structure. The first layer operates within the membrane, where vitamin E prevents the spread of lipid peroxidation at the point of initiation. The second layer operates at the interface, where glutathione-dependent enzymes reduce lipid peroxides that escape initial interception and prevent them from generating new radicals. The third layer operates through recycling, restoring oxidized components so they can continue to function. Each layer depends on the others. If vitamin E is depleted or not regenerated, more lipid radicals persist and place greater demand on glutathione. If glutathione is insufficient, the regeneration system slows and vitamin E remains in its inactive form, reducing protection within the membrane.

Lipid composition influences how this system performs. Membranes with a higher proportion of polyunsaturated fatty acids present more sites where lipid radicals can form. This increases reliance on vitamin E for immediate interception and on glutathione for downstream containment and regeneration. The balance between membrane composition and antioxidant capacity determines whether the system can maintain stability under ongoing reactive pressure. When these elements are aligned, reactive intermediates are contained within defined boundaries and membrane structure is preserved.

The interaction between glutathione, vitamin E, and lipid systems therefore functions as a coordinated network rather than separate protective mechanisms. Each component occupies a specific position and handles a defined part of the process, passing reactive load from one stage to the next until it is fully resolved. Stability depends on maintaining this sequence without interruption. When one part of the system slows or fails, the burden shifts to others, and the likelihood of propagation increases.

PART IV

FUNCTIONAL SYSTEMS

What glutathione actually does when embedded in biology

Chapter 9

Antioxidant Defense System

Antioxidant defense is not a collection of independent molecules acting in parallel. It is a coordinated system built to manage electron flow, contain reactive intermediates, and restore the structures altered during normal metabolism. Each component occupies a defined position within this system and performs a specific function that connects to the next step. The outcome depends on how these components interact, not on the presence of any single molecule in isolation. Glutathione sits at the center of this network because it links direct neutralization, enzymatic processing, and regeneration into a continuous cycle that can operate under sustained demand.

The system begins with the generation of reactive intermediates as a byproduct of energy production, substrate metabolism, and environmental exposure. These intermediates must be intercepted before they interact with cellular structures in an uncontrolled way. Enzymes such as superoxide dismutase convert highly reactive species into forms that can be further processed. Glutathione-dependent enzymes then take over, using reduced glutathione to convert peroxides and electrophilic compounds into stable products. This sequence does not eliminate reactivity at once. It transforms it step by step into forms that can be contained and removed without initiating secondary reactions.

Glutathione provides the core exchange mechanism that allows this sequence to function. Its ability to donate electrons and then be restored to its reduced form connects the initial interception of reactive intermediates with the recovery phase that maintains system capacity. When glutathione is available in sufficient amounts and recovery through NADPH-dependent pathways is intact, the system operates as a loop. Reactive intermediates are captured, converted, and resolved, and the molecules responsible for this process are returned to their active state. This prevents depletion and allows continuous operation under varying levels of demand.

Other components extend this system into different environments. Vitamin E operates within lipid membranes to intercept radicals at their point of origin. Vitamin C functions in the aqueous phase, supporting the regeneration of vitamin E and participating in direct reduction reactions. Enzymatic systems provide specificity, directing glutathione and other molecules toward defined substrates and pathways. These elements do not compete. They form a layered structure where each level handles a different stage of reactive processing, passing the intermediate from one component to the next until it is fully resolved.

The system is constrained by the availability of reducing equivalents, particularly NADPH, which drives the recovery phase. Without sufficient NADPH, oxidized glutathione accumulates and the capacity for further electron donation declines. This links antioxidant defense directly to metabolic pathways that generate reducing power, including those involved in glucose metabolism and cellular energy balance. When these pathways are functioning, recovery keeps pace with consumption. When they are limited, the system shifts toward accumulation of oxidized components and reduced buffering capacity.

Spatial organization determines how effectively this system operates within the cell. Different compartments maintain distinct antioxidant environments based on their specific demands. Mitochondria require rapid containment of continuously generated intermediates, while the cytosol provides broader stabilization across multiple pathways. Membrane systems rely on lipid-phase and aqueous-phase interactions to prevent propagation of peroxidation. These compartmental differences ensure that reactive intermediates are addressed at their point of origin rather than after they have spread.

Antioxidant defense therefore functions as a continuous process that transforms reactive intermediates into stable end products while preserving the molecules that perform this work. Glutathione integrates these steps by linking interception, containment, and recovery into a single cycle. Stability depends on maintaining this cycle across compartments and under varying levels of demand. When the system is intact, reactive intermediates are managed as part of normal metabolism. When it is disrupted, the same intermediates begin to accumulate and alter the structures that the system is designed to protect.

Reactive Oxygen Neutralization

Reactive oxygen species are generated continuously as electrons move through metabolic pathways, particularly within mitochondria, and their presence is not inherently abnormal. They become a problem when their lifetime extends beyond the narrow window in which they are meant to exist. Neutralization is the process of converting these intermediates into stable molecules before they interact with cellular structures, and this process occurs through a sequence of controlled reactions rather than a single step. Each stage reduces reactivity and passes the intermediate into a form that can be safely contained or removed.

The first stage involves conversion of highly reactive species into intermediates that can be handled by downstream systems. Superoxide dismutase converts superoxide into hydrogen peroxide, which is less reactive but still capable of initiating damage if it accumulates. This conversion concentrates reactive load into a form that can be processed more efficiently. Hydrogen peroxide can diffuse across compartments, making its control dependent on rapid interception before it reaches sensitive structures such as membranes or DNA.

Glutathione-dependent systems take over at this stage. Glutathione peroxidase uses reduced glutathione to convert hydrogen peroxide into water, removing its capacity to participate in further reactions. This reaction consumes reduced glutathione and produces its oxidized form, transferring the reactive burden into a contained state. The effectiveness of this step depends on maintaining a sufficient pool of reduced glutathione at the location where hydrogen peroxide is present. If this pool is depleted or recovery is delayed, hydrogen peroxide persists and begins to interact with lipids and proteins, initiating secondary reactions that extend beyond the original site of production.

Neutralization is therefore defined by timing and localization. Reactive intermediates must be intercepted at the point of formation or immediately after conversion into intermediate forms. Delay allows diffusion, increasing the number of potential targets and the likelihood of propagation. The system is designed to operate with minimal delay by maintaining high local concentrations of glutathione and the enzymes that use it. This ensures that reactive intermediates are resolved within the compartment where they are generated rather than after they have spread.

Recovery closes the cycle by restoring glutathione to its reduced form through glutathione reductase using NADPH. Without this step, neutralization would consume glutathione and reduce system capacity over time. Continuous recovery allows the same molecules to participate in repeated cycles, maintaining a stable buffering environment even under sustained reactive production. The rate of recovery must match the rate of neutralization to prevent accumulation of oxidized glutathione and loss of available thiol groups.

Reactive oxygen neutralization is not the elimination of reactive species from the system. It is the controlled conversion of these species into forms that no longer interact with cellular structures in a disruptive way. Glutathione anchors this process by linking interception, conversion, and recovery into a continuous cycle that operates at the scale and speed required to match ongoing metabolic activity.

Redox Buffering Capacity

Redox buffering capacity defines how much reactive load the cell can absorb without allowing that load to alter structure or function. It is not determined by the presence of glutathione alone but by the size of the reduced pool, the rate at which it can be regenerated, and how effectively it is distributed across compartments. The system operates as a standing reservoir of reducing equivalents that can be deployed immediately when reactive intermediates form. When this reservoir is sufficient, fluctuations in reactive production are contained within normal operating limits and do not propagate into structural change.

The reduced to oxidized glutathione ratio sets the baseline for this capacity. A high proportion of reduced glutathione means that most cysteine thiol groups are available to donate electrons, allowing rapid interception of reactive intermediates. As this ratio shifts toward the oxidized form, the number of available thiol groups declines, and the system becomes less responsive. The change is functional rather than symbolic. Fewer available electrons means slower containment, longer persistence of reactive intermediates, and a higher probability that these intermediates will interact with proteins, lipids, or DNA before being neutralized.

Capacity is also defined by recovery speed. Each time glutathione donates an electron, it moves into the oxidized state and must be reduced again to remain functional. Glutathione reductase, driven by NADPH, restores this state and returns the molecule to the active pool. If recovery matches consumption, the system maintains a steady supply of reduced glutathione even under increased demand. If recovery lags, the oxidized pool accumulates and the effective buffering capacity declines. This creates a condition where the total amount of glutathione may remain unchanged, but its functional availability is reduced.

Compartmental distribution shapes how this capacity is applied. The cytosol maintains a broad buffer that supports multiple pathways, while mitochondria require a tightly maintained local pool to manage continuous reactive production at the inner membrane. The nucleus depends on a stable redox environment to preserve DNA integrity and regulate transcription. Each compartment draws from the same underlying system but operates with different requirements for concentration and turnover. Capacity must therefore be sufficient not only in total but within each compartment where reactive intermediates are generated.

Demand is not constant. It increases with metabolic activity, exposure to external compounds, and shifts in substrate utilization. When demand rises within the limits of buffering capacity, the system absorbs the additional load and returns to baseline once conditions normalize.

When demand exceeds capacity, reactive intermediates persist, and the system begins to shift toward oxidation. This shift alters enzyme activity, membrane stability, and signaling behavior, creating changes that extend beyond the initial increase in reactive production.

Redox buffering capacity therefore represents the functional margin between controlled and uncontrolled reactivity. It is defined by how much disturbance the system can absorb while maintaining structure and function. Glutathione provides the central mechanism for this buffering, but its effectiveness depends on maintaining a high reduced pool, rapid recovery, and appropriate distribution. When these conditions are met, the cell operates within a stable redox range. When they are not, the system loses the ability to contain reactive intermediates and begins to accumulate changes that alter its internal environment.

Chapter 10

Detoxification Architecture

Detoxification is a structured process that converts reactive, lipophilic, or electrophilic compounds into forms that can be contained, transported, and eliminated. It is not a single reaction or pathway but a sequence of transformations that progressively change the chemical behavior of a compound. Each stage modifies how that compound interacts with cellular structures, reducing its ability to disrupt membranes, proteins, or DNA. Glutathione is integrated into this architecture at the point where reactive intermediates must be neutralized and prepared for removal, linking chemical transformation to physical clearance.

The first stage introduces or exposes reactive sites on compounds through oxidation, reduction, or hydrolysis. These reactions increase chemical reactivity rather than reducing it, creating intermediates that are easier to process but also more capable of interacting with cellular structures if left unresolved. This stage shifts the burden from recognition to containment. The cell must immediately direct these intermediates into controlled pathways or they will propagate damage. The output of this stage is therefore not a finished product but a substrate for further processing.

Glutathione enters at the stage where these intermediates are conjugated into stable forms. Through the action of glutathione S-transferases, glutathione binds to electrophilic compounds, forming conjugates that are less reactive and more water-compatible. This reaction neutralizes the electrophilic center that would otherwise interact with cellular components, effectively terminating its ability to participate in uncontrolled reactions. The resulting conjugate carries the compound in a form that can be recognized by transport systems and directed toward elimination.

This conjugation step depends on the availability of reduced glutathione. Each reaction consumes glutathione and transfers the reactive burden into a bound state. Recovery systems must restore glutathione to its reduced form to maintain capacity for continued detoxification. If supply or recovery is limited, reactive intermediates from earlier stages accumulate, increasing the likelihood that they will interact with unintended targets. The architecture therefore relies on continuous cycling rather than one-time use, maintaining throughput across the system.

After conjugation, compounds are moved through transport systems that direct them out of the cell or into compartments where further processing occurs. These transporters recognize the modified structure of glutathione conjugates and move them across membranes into bile, urine pathways, or extracellular space. The transformation carried out during conjugation is what allows this movement. Without it, many compounds would remain within lipid environments and continue interacting with cellular structures.

Detoxification architecture also includes recycling steps that recover components of glutathione after conjugates are processed. Enzymatic systems break down these conjugates outside the cell or in specific compartments, allowing amino acids to be reabsorbed and reused. This maintains substrate availability for continued glutathione synthesis and links detoxification back to amino acid metabolism. The system does not discard its components after use. It reclaims them to sustain ongoing function.

The entire process operates as a flow from activation to neutralization to elimination. Each stage depends on the one before it and sets the conditions for the one that follows. Glutathione provides the point where reactive intermediates are converted into stable, transportable forms, preventing them from interacting with cellular structures while enabling their removal. When this architecture is intact, compounds are processed and cleared without accumulating reactive burden. When it is disrupted, intermediates from early stages persist, increasing the risk of interaction with proteins, lipids, and DNA and shifting the system toward instability.

Phase I → Phase II → Conjugation

Detoxification proceeds as a sequence where each stage changes how a compound behaves inside the cell, and the transition between stages determines whether the process resolves safely or creates additional stress. Phase I introduces chemical modifications that expose or create reactive sites on a compound. These reactions, often carried out by enzyme systems that add oxygen or rearrange structure, increase the compound's ability to interact with other molecules. This does not neutralize it. It prepares it for the next step by making it more accessible, but at the same time increases the risk that it will react with cellular components if it is not immediately contained.

Phase II takes these reactive intermediates and attaches them to endogenous molecules that change their properties. Conjugation with glutathione is one of the primary mechanisms at this stage. The electrophilic center created during Phase I is bound by glutathione through the cysteine thiol, forming a stable conjugate that no longer seeks out proteins or lipids as reaction targets. This step converts a reactive intermediate into a controlled product that can be handled by transport systems. The transition from Phase I to Phase II must occur without delay. If conjugation capacity is insufficient, the intermediates generated in Phase I persist and begin to interact with surrounding structures, increasing cellular stress rather than resolving it.

Glutathione availability determines how effectively this transition is maintained. Each conjugation reaction consumes reduced glutathione, and recovery systems must restore it to sustain throughput. When the pool of reduced glutathione is sufficient, intermediates are rapidly bound and moved forward in the process. When it is limited, Phase I continues to generate reactive compounds that cannot be processed at the same rate, creating a mismatch between activation and containment. This mismatch shifts the system toward accumulation of reactive intermediates, which can bind to proteins or lipids in unintended ways.

Following conjugation, the modified compounds are directed toward elimination through transport systems that recognize their new structure. The addition of glutathione increases water compatibility and provides a signal for export, allowing these compounds to be moved out of the cell or into pathways that lead to excretion. The architecture depends on this final step to complete the process. Without effective transport, conjugated compounds would remain within the system and potentially undergo further reactions.

The sequence from Phase I through Phase II to elimination is therefore a continuous flow where each stage must match the output of the previous one. Phase I generates intermediates that must be immediately captured. Phase II, through glutathione conjugation, neutralizes and prepares them for removal. Transport systems complete the process by clearing them from the intracellular environment. Stability depends on maintaining balance across these stages. When they are aligned, compounds are processed and removed without accumulating reactive burden. When they are not, the system produces intermediates faster than it can resolve them, increasing the likelihood of interaction with cellular structures.

Glutathione Conjugation Pathways

Glutathione conjugation is the step where reactive intermediates are converted into stable, transportable forms, and this conversion is directed through enzyme systems that recognize specific chemical features rather than acting broadly on all substrates. Glutathione S-transferases provide the primary pathway for this process. These enzymes bind both glutathione and an electrophilic compound, positioning them so that the cysteine thiol can form a covalent bond with the reactive site. This reaction neutralizes the electrophilic center that would otherwise interact with proteins, lipids, or nucleic acids, effectively terminating its ability to propagate damage within the cell.

The pathway begins once a compound has been activated or exposed through earlier processing steps. Electrophilic intermediates present regions of electron deficiency that attract nucleophilic attack. The thiol group of glutathione serves as that nucleophile, forming a stable linkage that converts the intermediate into a conjugate. This transformation changes both reactivity and solubility. The compound no longer seeks out cellular structures as reaction partners, and its increased compatibility with aqueous environments allows it to be handled by transport systems. The reaction is not random. It is guided by enzyme specificity that determines which compounds are accepted and how efficiently the process proceeds.

Once formed, glutathione conjugates are directed toward export or further processing. Transport proteins recognize the modified structure and move these conjugates across membranes into bile, urine pathways, or extracellular space. This movement is an essential part of the pathway because the conjugate must be removed from the intracellular environment to complete detoxification. Retention within the cell would allow further reactions to occur, potentially reversing the stability achieved during conjugation.

The pathway extends beyond the initial conjugation step into a series of transformations that prepare the compound for final elimination. Outside the cell or within specific compartments, enzymes break down the glutathione portion of the conjugate, removing glutamate and glycine and leaving a cysteine-bound intermediate. This intermediate can then be further modified into a form that is more easily excreted. These downstream steps maintain the flow of the pathway while allowing recovery of amino acid components that can be reused for glutathione synthesis.

Throughput in this system depends on the availability of reduced glutathione and the activity of conjugating enzymes. Each reaction consumes glutathione, and recovery systems must regenerate it to sustain capacity. When glutathione supply is sufficient, the pathway operates continuously, converting reactive intermediates into stable products and moving them toward elimination. When supply is limited, intermediates accumulate and begin to interact with cellular structures before they can be conjugated. This shifts the system from controlled processing to uncontrolled interaction.

Glutathione conjugation pathways therefore function as a directed flow where reactive compounds are captured, transformed, and removed in a sequence that prevents their accumulation within the cell. The effectiveness of this flow depends on maintaining enzyme activity, substrate availability, and transport capacity in alignment. When these elements are coordinated, detoxification proceeds without disrupting cellular structure. When they are not, the same intermediates that are meant to be processed become sources of instability within the system.

Clearance vs Recirculation

Once a compound has been conjugated with glutathione, the system reaches a decision point that determines whether the process resolves or continues to cycle within the body. Clearance requires that the conjugate be moved out of the cell, transferred into bile or urine pathways, and ultimately eliminated. Recirculation occurs when this process is incomplete or reversed, allowing the compound or its derivatives to re-enter circulation and return to tissues. The difference between these outcomes is not defined by the initial detoxification step but by what happens after conjugation.

Transport systems govern the first stage of this decision. Glutathione conjugates are recognized by membrane transporters that move them out of the cell. This export depends on energy and functional transporter proteins embedded in cellular membranes. When these systems operate effectively, conjugated compounds are removed from the intracellular environment and directed toward excretory pathways. This lowers the local reactive burden and completes the detoxification sequence at the cellular level.

After export, the pathway continues through extracellular processing and organ-level handling. In the liver and bile system, conjugates can be secreted into bile and delivered to the intestine. From there, they may be excreted or further modified by enzymatic activity. In some cases, components of the conjugate are cleaved, producing derivatives that can be reabsorbed. This creates a loop where the compound re-enters circulation rather than being fully eliminated. The efficiency of clearance therefore depends on maintaining forward movement through this pathway without reversal.

Recirculation places additional demand on the detoxification system. Compounds that return to circulation must be processed again, consuming glutathione and enzymatic capacity each time they pass through the system. This repeated processing increases the overall load without reducing the total burden. The system continues to operate, but it does so under sustained demand that can exceed its capacity over time. As glutathione is consumed and recovery systems are taxed, the ability to manage new inputs declines.

The balance between clearance and recirculation is influenced by multiple factors, including transporter activity, enzymatic processing in downstream compartments, and the integrity of elimination pathways. When these systems are aligned, conjugated compounds move in a single direction toward removal, and the detoxification process reduces total burden. When they are not, compounds cycle back into the system, increasing exposure duration and amplifying demand on glutathione-dependent pathways.

This distinction determines whether detoxification functions as a resolving process or a repeating loop. Clearance reduces the presence of reactive compounds and restores system capacity. Recirculation maintains or increases the burden, requiring repeated use of the same resources without achieving resolution. The effectiveness of detoxification architecture therefore depends not only on the ability to conjugate reactive intermediates but on ensuring that those conjugates are carried through to final elimination without returning to the system.

Chapter 11

Immune Regulation

Immune function is governed by controlled activation and controlled resolution, and both phases depend on the redox environment within and around immune cells. Activation requires a shift toward a more oxidative state that allows signaling pathways to initiate, transcription factors to change configuration, and effector functions to engage. Resolution requires a return to a reduced state that terminates signaling, restores cellular structures, and prevents prolonged activation from damaging host tissue. Glutathione defines how precisely this transition occurs by setting the redox conditions that determine when immune responses begin, how strongly they proceed, and when they are brought back under control.

Immune cells generate reactive intermediates as part of their function, particularly during processes that target pathogens. These intermediates are used to alter or disrupt foreign structures, but they are produced within the same environment that contains host components. Containment is therefore required at the point of generation. Glutathione buffers this reactive output, allowing immune cells to produce sufficient reactive species to perform their function while preventing those species from spreading beyond their intended targets. The balance between production and containment determines whether the response remains localized or begins to affect surrounding tissue.

Redox state also influences signaling pathways that control immune activation. Transcription factors respond to changes in the intracellular environment by altering gene expression patterns that drive cytokine production, cell proliferation, and differentiation. These processes depend on reversible changes in protein structure that are sensitive to the ratio of reduced to oxidized glutathione. When the environment shifts toward oxidation, activation pathways are favored. When it returns toward reduction, those pathways are downregulated and the system moves toward resolution. Glutathione therefore acts as a control variable that shapes the duration and intensity of immune signaling.

The transition between activation and resolution must occur within defined limits. If the system remains in an oxidative state, signaling pathways continue to drive immune activity beyond what is required, leading to sustained inflammation and tissue damage. If the system shifts too quickly or too strongly toward reduction, activation may be insufficient to address the initiating stimulus. The immune system depends on maintaining a range where both phases can occur in sequence without overlap or delay. Glutathione availability and recovery determine how quickly the system can move between these states.

Compartmental dynamics further refine this control. Immune cells operate in environments where reactive production can be high and rapidly changing, requiring localized buffering that matches these fluctuations. At the same time, systemic signals must coordinate responses across tissues, linking local redox changes to broader immune behavior. Glutathione integrates these levels by maintaining intracellular stability while supporting the signaling mechanisms that communicate between cells.

Nutrient availability and metabolic state influence this regulation by determining the capacity to maintain glutathione levels and recovery. Amino acid supply, NADPH production, and overall cellular energy balance all contribute to the ability of immune cells to sustain controlled activation and resolution. When these inputs are sufficient, the system operates with precision. When they are limited, the transition between phases becomes less controlled, increasing the likelihood of prolonged activation or incomplete response.

Immune regulation therefore emerges from the ability to manage redox state within defined boundaries. Glutathione provides the mechanism that allows immune cells to generate reactive intermediates for functional purposes while preventing those intermediates from producing unintended damage. It also governs the signaling transitions that move the system from activation to resolution. When this control is intact, immune responses are targeted and self-limiting. When it is disrupted, the same processes that defend the system begin to alter it.

Activation vs Resolution

Immune activity begins with a shift in redox state that allows signaling pathways to engage and cellular functions to accelerate. This shift is not random. It is driven by localized changes in electron balance that alter protein configuration and enable transcription factors to initiate gene expression. Reactive intermediates increase during this phase, both as signaling tools and as direct effectors against external targets. The environment becomes more oxidative, which supports activation but also increases the risk of spillover into surrounding tissue if not contained. Glutathione does not prevent this shift. It sets the boundary within which activation can occur without becoming self-directed.

As activation progresses, immune cells produce reactive species in concentrated bursts. These species are used to alter or disrupt external structures, but they exist in the same physical space as host components. Containment depends on maintaining sufficient reduced glutathione to intercept excess intermediates that move beyond their intended targets. When this buffering capacity is intact, reactive output remains localized and temporary. When it is exceeded, intermediates persist and begin to interact with host proteins and membranes, extending the effect of activation beyond its intended scope.

Resolution requires a reversal of the redox conditions that supported activation. The system must return toward a reduced state so that signaling pathways disengage and cellular structures can be restored. Glutathione recovery becomes the dominant process in this phase, restoring protein thiols, reducing oxidized intermediates, and re-establishing baseline conditions. This transition is not passive. It depends on active reduction through NADPH-driven systems that return glutathione to its functional form. The speed and completeness of this recovery determine how quickly immune activity is brought back under control.

The timing between activation and resolution defines whether the response remains functional or becomes disruptive. If resolution follows activation within an appropriate window, reactive intermediates are cleared, signaling pathways shut down, and tissue integrity is preserved. If resolution is delayed, the oxidative environment persists, and the same mechanisms that were used for defense continue to operate without a defined target. This leads to ongoing interaction with host structures and progressive alteration of tissue.

Glutathione links these phases by controlling how far the system can move in either direction and how quickly it can return to baseline. During activation, it prevents reactive intermediates from exceeding the boundaries of the response. During resolution, it restores the environment required for normal cellular function. The system depends on maintaining both capacities simultaneously. If glutathione is insufficient, activation becomes less controlled and resolution becomes incomplete, creating overlap between phases where reactive processes continue without termination.

Activation and resolution are therefore not separate events but coordinated phases of a single process. The transition between them is governed by changes in redox state, and glutathione defines the limits and reversibility of those changes. When this control is intact, immune responses are targeted and self-limiting. When it is disrupted, the distinction between defense and damage begins to dissolve.

Inflammation Shutdown Capacity

Inflammation is initiated through signaling pathways that amplify local activity, recruit immune cells, and increase reactive output, but the system is only stable if it contains an equally defined mechanism for termination. Shutdown capacity refers to the ability to reverse the conditions that sustain inflammation and return the environment to baseline once the initiating stimulus has been addressed. This is not a passive decline. It requires active restoration of redox balance, structural repair, and disengagement of signaling pathways that were previously driving the response. Glutathione determines how effectively this transition occurs by controlling the redox conditions that allow inflammatory signaling to persist or resolve.

During active inflammation, the intracellular environment shifts toward oxidation. This state supports the activation of transcription factors and signaling proteins that drive cytokine production and maintain immune cell activity. As long as this environment is maintained, the system continues to operate in an activated mode. Shutdown requires reversing this shift. Reduced glutathione restores protein thiol groups that were altered during activation, returning signaling proteins to configurations that no longer support continued expression of inflammatory mediators. This change in protein structure directly reduces the signals that sustain the response.

Reactive intermediates produced during inflammation must also be cleared to complete the shutdown process. If they persist, they continue to interact with cellular structures and maintain the conditions that favor activation. Glutathione-dependent systems neutralize these intermediates and transfer the reactive burden into reversible forms that can be resolved through recovery pathways. The speed of this clearance determines how quickly the system can move out of the inflammatory state. Delayed clearance prolongs the presence of reactive intermediates, extending the duration of signaling and increasing the likelihood of tissue interaction.

Recovery of glutathione is central to this capacity. As inflammation progresses, reduced glutathione is consumed and converted into its oxidized form. Shutdown requires restoring this pool through NADPH-dependent reduction so that sufficient reducing equivalents are available to reverse oxidative changes. If recovery is incomplete, the system remains in a partially oxidized state, where some signaling pathways are still active and structural restoration is not fully achieved. This creates a condition where inflammation does not fully resolve but persists at a lower level, maintaining ongoing interaction with tissue.

Cellular and compartmental dynamics influence how shutdown capacity is distributed. Immune cells operating at the site of inflammation require rapid local restoration, while surrounding tissues depend on a broader return to baseline conditions. Glutathione must be sufficient in both contexts to ensure that resolution occurs not only at the site of activation but across the affected system. A localized deficit can prolong activity in one region even if overall conditions appear to improve.

When shutdown capacity is intact, inflammation proceeds as a defined sequence with a clear endpoint. Activation occurs, the initiating stimulus is addressed, and the system returns to baseline conditions without residual activity. When this capacity is limited, the system remains partially activated, with ongoing signaling and reactive production that continue to alter tissue over time. The distinction between acute and persistent inflammation is therefore determined by the ability to restore redox balance and terminate signaling within an appropriate timeframe. Glutathione provides the mechanism that enables this transition, defining whether the inflammatory response resolves or continues.

Chapter 12

Cellular Repair and Survival

Cellular repair is not a separate process that begins after damage occurs. It operates continuously alongside metabolism, correcting structural changes as they arise and maintaining the integrity of proteins, membranes, and genetic material. Survival depends on how effectively the cell can identify altered structures, reverse those alterations, and restore function before damage accumulates beyond repairable limits. Glutathione is embedded in this process at the level where chemical changes first appear, controlling whether those changes remain reversible or progress into structural loss.

Proteins are particularly sensitive to changes in redox state because their function depends on maintaining specific three-dimensional configurations. Reactive intermediates can alter amino acid residues, especially those containing sulfur groups, changing how the protein folds and interacts with other molecules. Glutathione participates directly in reversing these changes by restoring thiol groups to their reduced state, allowing proteins to return to their functional configuration. This is not a one-time correction. It occurs repeatedly as proteins cycle through states of use, exposure, and restoration. When this process is maintained, enzyme systems remain active and structural proteins retain their integrity.

Membrane repair follows a similar principle but operates through containment and replacement rather than direct reversal of individual molecular changes. When lipid peroxidation is initiated, glutathione-dependent systems terminate the propagation of damage, limiting the affected area. This containment prevents widespread disruption and allows localized repair processes to replace altered lipids without compromising the entire membrane structure. The effectiveness of this process depends on stopping the chain reaction early. Once propagation spreads beyond a limited region, repair requires larger-scale restructuring that carries greater functional cost.

DNA stability depends on maintaining a controlled environment where reactive intermediates do not persist long enough to alter nucleotide structure. Glutathione supports this by maintaining a reduced nuclear environment and by participating in systems that resolve oxidative modifications before they become fixed changes. When reactive intermediates are contained quickly, DNA integrity is preserved and normal replication and transcription proceed. When they persist, the likelihood of permanent alteration increases, shifting the system from repair toward accumulated change.

Cellular survival is determined by the balance between damage and repair capacity. When glutathione levels are sufficient and recovery systems are intact, the cell can continuously reverse chemical alterations and maintain structural integrity under normal metabolic conditions. When this balance shifts, and reactive load exceeds the capacity for containment and repair, alterations begin to accumulate. Proteins lose function, membranes become unstable, and genetic material becomes more susceptible to change. The system moves from a state of controlled maintenance to one where structural degradation progresses.

Energy availability influences this balance by determining the resources available for repair processes. Many repair mechanisms require ATP and reducing equivalents, linking cellular survival to overall metabolic state. Glutathione connects these requirements by using NADPH for recovery and by supporting the enzymatic systems that carry out repair. When energy production is stable, repair processes can operate continuously. When it is impaired, recovery slows and the system becomes less capable of reversing damage.

Repair and survival are therefore not independent outcomes but part of the same continuous process. The cell survives by maintaining the ability to reverse chemical changes as they occur, preventing them from progressing into structural failure. Glutathione provides the mechanism that keeps these changes within a reversible range, allowing the system to maintain function over time. When this mechanism is intact, cellular structures are preserved despite ongoing metabolic activity. When it is compromised, the accumulation of unresolved changes shifts the system toward loss of function and reduced viability.

DNA Protection

DNA exists in a state that is chemically stable but constantly exposed to reactive intermediates generated by normal cellular activity. These intermediates can alter nucleotide bases, disrupt the sugar backbone, or interfere with proteins that control replication and transcription. Protection is not achieved by isolating DNA from these influences, because reactive species are produced within the same compartment. It is achieved by controlling how long these intermediates persist and how far they can diffuse before being neutralized. Glutathione defines this control by maintaining a nuclear environment where reactive species are resolved before they interact with genetic material.

The nuclear redox state determines how susceptible DNA is to modification. A reduced environment keeps reactive intermediates in check and preserves the structure of both DNA and the proteins that regulate it. When this environment shifts toward oxidation, reactive intermediates persist longer and increase the probability of interaction with nucleotide bases. These interactions can alter base pairing or create structural irregularities that interfere with replication and transcription. Glutathione maintains the reduced state required to limit these interactions, ensuring that reactive intermediates are converted into stable forms before they reach DNA.

Protection also extends to the proteins that organize and interpret genetic material. Transcription factors and repair enzymes rely on specific structural configurations that are sensitive to redox conditions. Oxidative changes can alter these configurations, reducing their ability to bind DNA or carry out repair functions. Glutathione restores these proteins to their functional state by reducing altered thiol groups, allowing them to maintain control over gene expression and correction of structural changes. This indirect protection is essential because DNA stability depends not only on the molecule itself but on the systems that manage it.

When reactive intermediates are not contained, they can produce modifications that require active repair. Cellular repair systems identify and remove altered bases, replacing them with correct structures to maintain genetic integrity. The effectiveness of these systems depends on both energy availability and redox conditions. Glutathione supports this process by maintaining an environment where repair enzymes can function and by limiting the number of modifications that need to be addressed. When the rate of damage exceeds the capacity for repair, alterations accumulate and begin to affect how genetic information is used.

Compartmental interaction influences how this protection is maintained. The nuclear environment is linked to the cytosolic and mitochondrial redox states, and changes in one compartment can affect conditions in another. Increased reactive production in mitochondria, for example, can extend into the cytosol and influence nuclear conditions if not contained. Glutathione distribution across these compartments ensures that local increases in reactive load do not propagate into the nucleus.

DNA protection therefore depends on maintaining a controlled redox environment that limits exposure to reactive intermediates and supports the systems responsible for repair and regulation. Glutathione provides the mechanism that keeps these conditions within a range where genetic material remains stable and functional. When this control is intact, DNA is preserved despite continuous metabolic activity. When it is disrupted, the likelihood of structural alteration increases, shifting the system from maintenance toward accumulated change.

Protein Preservation

Proteins operate through precise three-dimensional structures that depend on the chemical state of their constituent amino acids. Many of these amino acids contain groups that can be altered by reactive intermediates, changing how the protein folds, binds, or catalyzes reactions. These alterations do not always destroy the protein immediately. They shift it into a different configuration, often reducing efficiency or changing specificity. Preservation depends on keeping these changes within a reversible range and restoring the original structure before the protein is marked for degradation or replaced.

Glutathione maintains this reversibility by controlling the redox state of cysteine residues within proteins. These residues can form disulfide bonds under oxidative conditions, altering the shape of the protein and its interaction with other molecules. When glutathione is available in its reduced form, it restores these residues to their original state, breaking inappropriate disulfide bonds and returning the protein to its functional configuration. This process occurs continuously as proteins cycle through exposure to reactive intermediates and subsequent restoration. The system does not prevent all modification. It ensures that modification does not become permanent.

Reactive intermediates can also produce more extensive changes when they persist, including oxidation of amino acid side chains or fragmentation of protein structure. These changes move beyond reversible shifts and require removal of the affected protein. Glutathione limits the progression to this stage by intercepting reactive intermediates before they interact extensively with protein surfaces. When containment is effective, most interactions remain at the level of reversible thiol modification. When containment fails, proteins accumulate irreversible changes and must be degraded and replaced, increasing metabolic cost and reducing functional capacity during the transition.

Protein preservation is closely linked to enzymatic activity. Enzymes depend on active sites that require precise chemical conditions to bind substrates and carry out reactions. Small changes in redox state can alter these sites, reducing catalytic efficiency or preventing the reaction entirely. Glutathione maintains the environment required for these sites to remain functional, allowing metabolic pathways to proceed without interruption. When this control is lost, enzyme activity declines across multiple pathways, creating system-wide effects that extend beyond individual proteins.

The balance between preservation and turnover determines how the cell manages its protein pool. When glutathione-mediated restoration is sufficient, proteins are maintained and reused, conserving resources and maintaining continuity of function. When restoration is insufficient, damaged proteins accumulate and are targeted for degradation, requiring increased synthesis to replace them. This shift increases demand on amino acid supply and energy production, linking protein preservation to broader metabolic capacity.

Compartmental differences influence how this process is managed. In environments with higher reactive production, such as mitochondria, the demand for rapid restoration is greater, and local glutathione availability becomes critical. In the cytosol, where proteins from multiple pathways interact, maintaining a stable redox environment supports coordinated function across systems. The nucleus relies on preservation of regulatory proteins that control gene expression, linking protein stability to cellular behavior at a higher level.

Protein preservation therefore depends on maintaining a redox environment that keeps structural changes reversible and prevents progression to irreversible damage. Glutathione provides the mechanism that restores altered residues, supports enzyme function, and limits the accumulation of damaged proteins. When this system is intact, proteins retain their structure and function despite continuous exposure to reactive intermediates. When it is compromised, structural alterations accumulate and shift the balance toward increased turnover and reduced efficiency.

Apoptosis vs Recovery Decisions

Cells do not respond to stress in a binary way. They continuously assess whether structural changes remain within a reversible range or have progressed beyond the point where normal function can be restored. This assessment is carried out through signals that reflect redox state, energy availability, and the extent of molecular damage. Glutathione sits at the center of this evaluation because it determines whether reactive intermediates are being contained and reversed or whether they are accumulating and altering core structures. The decision to continue repair or initiate programmed cell death emerges from this balance.

When glutathione levels are sufficient and recovery systems are operating, most oxidative changes remain reversible. Proteins can be restored to their functional state, membrane damage is contained before it spreads, and DNA alterations are limited to levels that repair systems can correct. Under these conditions, signaling pathways favor survival. The cell maintains mitochondrial integrity, preserves membrane potential, and continues to produce energy required for repair processes. The environment remains within a range where restoration is energetically and structurally feasible.

As reactive load increases and glutathione becomes depleted or remains in its oxidized form, the system shifts. Reactive intermediates persist longer and begin to produce changes that cannot be reversed through standard repair mechanisms. Mitochondrial membranes become more permeable, disrupting the gradient required for energy production. Protein structures accumulate irreversible modifications, and DNA damage exceeds the capacity of repair systems to correct it accurately. These changes generate signals that indicate loss of structural integrity rather than temporary disruption.

Mitochondria play a central role in this transition because they integrate both energy status and redox signals. When glutathione-dependent protection within the mitochondria fails, reactive intermediates alter membrane structure and disrupt electron transport. This reduces ATP output and increases further reactive production, creating a self-reinforcing condition. As membrane integrity declines, signaling molecules that initiate apoptosis are released into the cytosol. This marks a shift from a system attempting repair to one that is actively dismantling itself in a controlled manner.

The decision point is therefore not a single trigger but a threshold where cumulative changes alter the signaling environment. High levels of reduced glutathione support pathways that maintain mitochondrial function, suppress apoptotic signaling, and favor repair. As the ratio shifts toward oxidation and structural damage accumulates, these survival signals weaken and apoptotic pathways become dominant. The system moves toward containment of damage at the organismal level by removing the compromised cell.

Energy availability influences this decision because repair requires sustained ATP production and reducing equivalents. When energy production is maintained, the cell has the resources to restore altered structures and recover from transient stress. When mitochondrial function declines, the capacity to support repair diminishes, and the system favors termination over incomplete restoration. Glutathione connects these factors by maintaining mitochondrial stability and supporting the recovery processes that depend on NADPH.

Apoptosis and recovery are therefore outcomes of the same underlying evaluation. The cell measures whether it can restore its internal environment to a stable state or whether continued operation would propagate dysfunction. Glutathione defines the boundary of this decision by controlling the extent and reversibility of oxidative changes. When its buffering and recovery capacity are sufficient, the system remains in a repair mode. When they are exceeded, the balance shifts toward programmed cell death as a means of preserving the integrity of the larger system.

PART V

SYNTHESIS → RECYCLING → AVAILABILITY

Why levels rise or fall

Chapter 13

Glutathione Synthesis

Glutathione synthesis is a controlled, multi-step process that determines how much buffering capacity the cell can maintain at any given time. It is not a passive reflection of amino acid availability but an energy-dependent sequence that integrates substrate supply, enzymatic control, and cellular demand. The system builds glutathione in the cytosol through two sequential reactions, each requiring ATP, and each sensitive to the current redox state. This creates a feedback structure where synthesis increases when demand rises and slows when sufficient levels are present.

The first step combines glutamate and cysteine through the enzyme glutamate-cysteine ligase, forming a gamma-linked intermediate that defines the structure of glutathione. This step sets the rate of the entire pathway because it depends on cysteine availability and is subject to inhibition by existing glutathione levels. When reduced glutathione is abundant, the enzyme slows its activity, preventing unnecessary accumulation. When glutathione is consumed and the pool shifts toward oxidation, this inhibition is relieved, allowing synthesis to increase. The system therefore adjusts production based on how much buffering capacity remains available.

Cysteine availability determines whether this step can proceed at the required rate. Unlike glutamate, which is widely available, cysteine is limited and must be supplied through diet or generated through conversion pathways that depend on other nutrients. When cysteine is sufficient, the system can respond to increased demand by accelerating synthesis. When it is limited, the pathway cannot scale, and glutathione levels become constrained regardless of demand. This establishes a direct link between sulfur amino acid metabolism and the capacity to maintain redox balance.

The second step adds glycine to the intermediate through glutathione synthetase, completing the tripeptide structure. This step is less tightly regulated but still depends on substrate availability and energy input. Glycine must be available in sufficient amounts to sustain production, and its allocation across competing pathways influences how efficiently this step proceeds. While not typically rate-limiting, insufficient glycine can reduce overall throughput when demand for glutathione increases.

Energy input is required for both steps, linking synthesis to the overall metabolic state of the cell. ATP availability determines how quickly these reactions can proceed, and NADPH indirectly influences synthesis by maintaining the reduced state that signals demand. When energy production is stable, synthesis can increase to meet rising reactive load. When energy is limited, the system cannot expand production even if demand is high, creating a condition where consumption exceeds replenishment.

Synthesis operates alongside recycling rather than replacing it. The majority of glutathione function is maintained through the reduction of oxidized glutathione back to its active form. Synthesis provides the additional capacity required when demand exceeds what recycling alone can sustain. The balance between these processes determines whether the total glutathione pool expands, contracts, or remains stable over time.

Transport and compartmental distribution depend on this cytosolic synthesis. Glutathione produced in the cytosol supplies other compartments, including mitochondria, which rely on import rather than local production. This makes cytosolic synthesis a central point of control for the entire system. A reduction in synthesis affects not only the cytosolic pool but also the ability to maintain glutathione levels across compartments with distinct demands.

Glutathione synthesis therefore defines the upper limit of buffering capacity. It determines how much the system can expand in response to increased reactive load and how quickly depleted pools can be restored. When substrate availability, energy input, and enzymatic regulation are aligned, synthesis supports continuous adaptation to changing conditions. When any of these factors are constrained, the system loses the ability to maintain its pool, and buffering capacity declines despite ongoing demand.

Rate-Limiting Role of Cysteine

Cysteine determines how much glutathione the cell can produce because it is the least available and most tightly controlled substrate in the synthesis pathway. Glutamate and glycine are broadly present and can be drawn from multiple metabolic pools, but cysteine exists in a more restricted supply and is actively regulated due to its chemical reactivity. The first step of glutathione synthesis requires cysteine to combine with glutamate, and if cysteine is not available at that moment, the pathway cannot proceed regardless of how much of the other substrates are present. This places cysteine at the point where production is either enabled or halted.

The limitation is structural and metabolic at the same time. Cysteine contains a sulfur group that gives glutathione its reactive capacity, but that same feature makes free cysteine potentially disruptive if it accumulates. The cell therefore maintains it at low concentrations, storing or converting it into other forms when not immediately needed. This protective control reduces the risk of uncontrolled reactions but creates a bottleneck when demand for glutathione increases. The system cannot simply draw from a large reserve. It must generate or import cysteine in real time to support synthesis.

Cysteine supply depends on both external input and internal conversion pathways. Dietary protein provides cysteine directly or through methionine, which can be converted into cysteine through sulfur transfer pathways that require additional nutrients and enzymatic steps. When these inputs are sufficient, cysteine availability supports steady glutathione production and allows the system to respond to increased demand. When they are limited, synthesis slows, and the total glutathione pool begins to reflect that constraint. This creates a direct link between sulfur amino acid metabolism and redox buffering capacity.

As glutathione is consumed during periods of increased reactive load, the need for cysteine rises. If supply cannot match this increased demand, the system shifts toward reliance on recycling existing glutathione rather than expanding the pool. This can maintain function temporarily, but it reduces the ability to handle sustained or escalating stress. Over time, the imbalance between consumption and synthesis leads to a decline in available reduced glutathione, even if recovery systems remain active.

The rate-limiting role of cysteine also influences how quickly the system can recover after depletion. Once glutathione levels fall, restoring them requires sufficient cysteine to rebuild the pool. If cysteine supply remains constrained, recovery is prolonged, and the system operates with reduced buffering capacity for an extended period. This delays the return to a stable redox environment and increases the likelihood that reactive intermediates will persist during that interval.

Cysteine therefore defines the ceiling and recovery speed of glutathione synthesis. It controls whether the system can scale production to meet demand and how quickly it can restore capacity after depletion. When cysteine availability is aligned with metabolic needs, glutathione synthesis supports stable redox control. When it is not, the entire system becomes constrained at the level of substrate supply, limiting the cell's ability to maintain internal stability under changing conditions.

Rate-Limiting Role of Glycine

Glycine does not control the entry point into glutathione synthesis in the same way cysteine does, but it determines whether the pathway can complete and sustain output once it has started. The final step of synthesis requires glycine to be added to the gamma-linked glutamate–cysteine intermediate, forming the finished tripeptide. If glycine is not available at that moment, the intermediate accumulates but cannot be converted into functional glutathione. This creates a secondary bottleneck where the system initiates synthesis but fails to produce usable output at the rate required to maintain buffering capacity.

The limitation emerges from competition across multiple pathways that draw from the same glycine pool. Glycine is used for protein synthesis, collagen formation, heme production, and one-carbon metabolism, where it supports methylation reactions and nucleotide synthesis. These processes operate continuously and increase their demand under conditions of growth, repair, or high metabolic activity. As demand in these pathways rises, less glycine is available to complete glutathione synthesis. The system does not prioritize one pathway automatically. Allocation is determined by immediate metabolic pressures, which means glutathione production can be constrained even when the need for redox buffering is high.

Unlike cysteine, which is tightly regulated due to its reactivity, glycine is more freely distributed but more widely consumed. This creates a different type of bottleneck. The limitation is not caused by restricted availability in absolute terms but by dilution of supply across competing uses. When glycine demand is balanced, the synthesis pathway proceeds without interruption and supports steady glutathione production. When demand increases in other systems, the throughput of glutathione synthesis declines, reducing the rate at which new molecules enter the pool.

This constraint becomes more apparent under sustained stress. As glutathione is consumed and must be replaced, the requirement for glycine rises alongside cysteine. If glycine supply does not scale with this demand, the system cannot fully replenish its pool even if the first step of synthesis continues to operate. The result is a gradual reduction in total glutathione availability, not because the pathway is inactive, but because it is incomplete at the final stage.

Energy and metabolic state influence this role as well. Glycine participates in pathways that are directly tied to cellular growth and repair, and increased activity in these areas can redirect glycine away from glutathione synthesis. This links the completion of glutathione production to broader physiological priorities, where the system must balance structural demands with the need to maintain redox stability.

Glycine therefore defines the throughput of glutathione synthesis once the pathway has been initiated. It determines whether intermediate structures are converted into functional molecules at a rate that matches consumption. When glycine is sufficient relative to competing demands, the system maintains a stable supply of glutathione. When it is not, synthesis becomes incomplete, and buffering capacity declines despite ongoing activity in earlier steps of the pathway.

Enzymatic Construction

Glutathione is assembled through a defined enzymatic sequence that controls both the structure of the molecule and the rate at which it enters the cellular pool. This construction does not occur spontaneously. It requires two ATP-dependent reactions that link specific amino acids in a configuration that standard peptide assembly does not produce. The enzymes involved determine when synthesis occurs, how fast it proceeds, and how the system responds to changes in demand.

The first step is carried out by glutamate-cysteine ligase, which joins glutamate and cysteine through the gamma-glutamyl bond. This reaction establishes the structural feature that protects glutathione from rapid degradation and allows it to persist within the cell. The enzyme operates under feedback control, responding to the existing concentration of glutathione. When levels are high, the enzyme slows, limiting additional production. When glutathione is consumed and the pool shifts toward oxidation, this inhibition is reduced, allowing synthesis to increase. This creates a direct link between current buffering capacity and production rate.

The formation of this intermediate requires ATP, which provides the energy needed to create a bond that does not form under normal conditions. This ties synthesis to the energy state of the cell. When ATP is available, the reaction proceeds efficiently. When energy is limited, the rate of construction declines regardless of substrate availability. The system therefore integrates structural assembly with metabolic capacity, ensuring that production does not exceed what the cell can support.

The second step is carried out by glutathione synthetase, which adds glycine to the intermediate to complete the tripeptide. This reaction finalizes the molecule, producing a structure that can participate in redox buffering, detoxification, and transport processes. While this step is less tightly regulated than the first, it still depends on substrate availability and ATP input. If glycine is limited or energy is constrained, the intermediate cannot be converted into functional glutathione at the required rate.

These two steps form a continuous construction pathway where initiation and completion must remain aligned. If the first step proceeds without sufficient capacity in the second, intermediates accumulate without increasing functional output. If the second step is ready but the first is limited by cysteine availability or feedback inhibition, overall production remains constrained. The system maintains balance by adjusting enzyme activity based on substrate levels and current glutathione concentration.

Enzymatic construction operates alongside recycling systems that restore oxidized glutathione to its reduced form. Synthesis provides new molecules when demand exceeds what recycling can sustain, expanding the total pool rather than simply maintaining it. This distinction becomes critical under sustained stress, where both construction and recovery must operate together to prevent depletion.

The structure produced through this enzymatic sequence defines how glutathione behaves within the cell. The gamma-glutamyl bond protects it from degradation, the cysteine thiol provides the reactive center for electron exchange, and the glycine residue contributes to mobility and interaction with transport systems. Each step in construction establishes a feature that is required for function, linking the process of synthesis directly to the role the molecule plays once it is formed.Nutrient dependencies

Chapter 14

Recycling Systems

Glutathione function depends more on recycling than on synthesis. Each time it donates an electron or forms a conjugate, it moves into a state that is no longer immediately usable. If the system relied only on new synthesis to replace this loss, the metabolic cost would be too high and the response too slow to match ongoing demand. Recycling restores glutathione to its active form within the same cellular space and timeframe in which it was used, allowing the system to maintain a stable pool that can respond continuously to reactive load.

The core of this system is the conversion of oxidized glutathione back into its reduced form. When two glutathione molecules form a disulfide bond, they store reactive load in a controlled configuration. Glutathione reductase reverses this bond using NADPH as the electron source, regenerating two molecules of reduced glutathione. This reaction closes the redox cycle, returning glutathione to a state where it can again donate electrons. The rate of this conversion determines whether the system maintains a high proportion of reduced glutathione or shifts toward accumulation of the oxidized form.

NADPH supply sets the capacity of this recycling process. It provides the reducing power required to restore glutathione and is generated through metabolic pathways that operate alongside energy production and biosynthesis. When NADPH production is sufficient, recycling keeps pace with consumption and the system maintains a stable redox environment. When it is limited, oxidized glutathione accumulates and the availability of reduced molecules declines, reducing the system's ability to intercept new reactive intermediates.

Recycling extends beyond redox conversion into the recovery of glutathione components after detoxification. When glutathione conjugates are formed and exported, enzymatic systems outside the cell or in specialized compartments break them down into their constituent amino acids. These components can then be reabsorbed and used to rebuild glutathione, linking detoxification pathways back to synthesis. This recovery prevents loss of substrate and supports sustained production under continuous demand.

Compartmental dynamics influence how recycling is maintained. The cytosol supports the majority of glutathione reductase activity, maintaining the central pool that supplies other regions. Mitochondria rely on localized recycling to sustain their internal glutathione levels, as direct replacement from the cytosol is limited. Each compartment must therefore maintain its own balance between oxidation and reduction to prevent localized depletion.

The efficiency of recycling determines how the system responds to sustained or increasing reactive load. When recycling matches or exceeds consumption, glutathione remains available and the system maintains control over redox conditions. When consumption outpaces recycling, the pool shifts toward oxidation, and the system loses its ability to contain reactive intermediates effectively. This shift occurs even if total glutathione levels remain unchanged, because functional capacity depends on the proportion that is in the reduced state.

Recycling systems therefore define the continuity of glutathione function. They allow the same molecules to participate in repeated cycles of electron donation and recovery, maintaining a stable buffering environment without requiring constant replacement. When these systems are intact, glutathione operates as a persistent component of cellular architecture. When they are impaired, the system becomes dependent on slower synthesis pathways and begins to lose its ability to respond to ongoing metabolic activity.

Glutathione Reductase

Glutathione reductase maintains the functional state of the glutathione pool by converting oxidized glutathione back into its reduced form. When glutathione donates electrons, two molecules link through a disulfide bond and move into a state that cannot participate in further reactions until it is reversed. Glutathione reductase performs that reversal. It uses electrons supplied by NADPH to break the disulfide bond and restore two active molecules, each with a free thiol group ready to engage reactive intermediates again. This reaction is continuous and operates at the same scale as glutathione consumption, ensuring that the system maintains a high proportion of reduced glutathione under normal conditions.

The activity of this enzyme defines whether the redox system remains functional or begins to shift toward accumulation of oxidized forms. When glutathione reductase operates efficiently and NADPH supply is sufficient, oxidized glutathione is rapidly converted back into its reduced state. The pool remains predominantly active, and reactive intermediates are intercepted as they are generated. When this process slows, oxidized glutathione accumulates and the number of available thiol groups declines. The system does not lose glutathione in total, but it loses the portion that can actively participate in electron transfer, reducing its capacity to contain reactive load.

NADPH availability sets the rate at which glutathione reductase can function. The enzyme itself may be present and capable, but without a continuous supply of reducing equivalents, it cannot restore oxidized glutathione at the required rate. This links glutathione recycling directly to metabolic pathways that generate NADPH. When these pathways are active, the enzyme maintains a steady flow of reduction. When they are constrained, recovery slows and the balance between reduced and oxidized forms shifts toward oxidation.

Compartmental distribution affects how this process supports different regions of the cell. In the cytosol, glutathione reductase maintains the primary pool that supplies other compartments. In mitochondria, local recycling is required to sustain the internal glutathione environment, as reliance on cytosolic import alone is insufficient for immediate demand.

Each compartment depends on maintaining sufficient enzyme activity and NADPH supply to preserve its own redox conditions.

The relationship between glutathione reductase and reactive load is dynamic. Increased production of reactive intermediates leads to increased oxidation of glutathione, which in turn requires increased activity of the enzyme to restore balance. If the enzyme and NADPH supply scale with this demand, the system maintains stability. If they do not, oxidized glutathione accumulates and reactive intermediates begin to persist, marking the transition toward reduced buffering capacity.

Glutathione reductase therefore functions as the recovery engine of the redox system. It determines how quickly the system can return to a state where glutathione is available for further reactions. Without this continuous restoration, glutathione would shift into an inactive form and the cell would lose its ability to manage reactive intermediates effectively. The enzyme does not increase total glutathione, but it preserves its functional state, allowing the system to operate as a continuous cycle rather than a one-time consumption process.

NADPH Dependence

Glutathione recycling is limited by the availability of reducing equivalents, and NADPH provides the electron supply that drives this process. When glutathione becomes oxidized, it cannot return to its active form without receiving electrons. Glutathione reductase performs the conversion, but it depends entirely on NADPH to supply those electrons. This creates a direct dependency where the capacity to restore glutathione is not determined by the amount of enzyme present but by how much NADPH the cell can generate and maintain.

NADPH is produced through metabolic pathways that operate alongside energy production, but its role is distinct. It is not used to generate ATP. It is reserved for reductive processes that maintain cellular structure and chemical balance. This includes recycling glutathione, supporting biosynthesis, and maintaining the reduced state of other critical molecules. When NADPH production is sufficient, oxidized glutathione is rapidly converted back into its reduced form, preserving the pool of active molecules required for continuous buffering. When

NADPH is limited, this conversion slows, and oxidized glutathione begins to accumulate.

The rate of NADPH generation sets the ceiling for how much reactive load the system can handle. As reactive intermediates are neutralized, glutathione is consumed and must be restored. Each cycle requires NADPH. If reactive production increases, demand for NADPH rises in parallel. If supply does not match this increase, the system reaches a point where recycling cannot keep pace with consumption. Reduced glutathione declines, and reactive intermediates persist longer within the cell, increasing the likelihood of interaction with structural components.

This dependency links redox control to broader metabolic state. Pathways that generate NADPH must remain active to support glutathione recycling. When these pathways are functioning, the system maintains a steady flow of reducing equivalents that sustain recovery. When they are impaired or redirected, the supply of NADPH becomes constrained, and the ability to restore glutathione declines even if total glutathione levels remain unchanged.

Compartmental demands further refine this relationship. Mitochondria require localized reducing power to maintain their internal glutathione pool, while the cytosol supports a broader distribution. Each compartment must generate or receive sufficient NADPH to sustain its own recycling processes. A deficit in one area can lead to localized accumulation of oxidized glutathione, even if overall cellular NADPH appears adequate.

NADPH dependence therefore defines the recovery capacity of the glutathione system. It determines how quickly oxidized glutathione can be returned to its active state and how long the system can sustain continuous neutralization of reactive intermediates. When NADPH supply matches demand, the system operates as a closed cycle with stable buffering capacity. When it does not, the cycle slows, and the balance shifts toward oxidation, reducing the cell's ability to maintain internal stability under ongoing metabolic activity.

Continuous Reuse vs Depletion

Glutathione operates as a reusable component of cellular architecture rather than a disposable antioxidant. Each time it donates an electron, it enters an oxidized state that can be restored and returned to function through the action of glutathione reductase and the availability of NADPH. This creates a closed cycle where the same molecules move repeatedly between reduced and oxidized states, handling reactive load without being permanently consumed. When this cycle remains intact, the total glutathione pool does not need to expand continuously because the existing molecules are used, recovered, and reused at a rate that matches demand.

Continuous reuse depends on alignment between three processes: oxidation, reduction, and energy supply. Reactive intermediates drive oxidation of glutathione. Glutathione reductase reverses that oxidation. NADPH provides the electrons required for the reversal. When these processes remain synchronized, glutathione cycles rapidly between states, and the proportion of reduced molecules stays high. The system maintains a stable buffer that absorbs reactive fluctuations without requiring large changes in total glutathione levels.

Depletion begins when this alignment breaks. If reactive production increases beyond what recycling can handle, more glutathione is pushed into the oxidized state than can be restored in the same timeframe. If NADPH supply is limited, the reduction step slows even if enzyme activity remains intact. If synthesis cannot add new molecules quickly enough to compensate, the pool shifts toward oxidation and the amount of available reduced glutathione declines. The system still contains glutathione, but a larger portion of it is no longer in a form that can actively participate in electron transfer.

A second layer of depletion occurs when glutathione is diverted into pathways that remove it from the cycle entirely. During detoxification, glutathione forms conjugates that are exported out of the cell. These molecules are not immediately available for recycling. They must be broken down and their components recovered before they can contribute to new synthesis. This creates a loss of immediate buffering capacity, especially when conjugation rates increase under high chemical load.

The transition from reuse to depletion is gradual rather than abrupt. Early on, the system compensates through increased recycling and modest increases in synthesis. As demand continues or intensifies, the gap between consumption and recovery widens. Reduced glutathione declines, oxidized forms accumulate, and reactive intermediates persist longer within the cell. This shift alters how the system behaves, moving from rapid containment to delayed response.

Continuous reuse maintains stability by keeping glutathione in its active form and within the cell. Depletion reflects a failure of recovery processes to match consumption, either through insufficient NADPH, impaired enzymatic activity, or diversion of glutathione into export pathways. The balance between these states determines whether the glutathione system functions as a sustained buffer or begins to lose capacity under ongoing metabolic pressure.

Chapter 15

System Bottlenecks

Glutathione capacity is not determined by a single variable but by the alignment of multiple inputs that must operate together without interruption. The system depends on substrate availability, enzymatic throughput, energy supply, and reducing equivalents. When these components are balanced, glutathione functions as a continuous cycle with stable buffering capacity. When any one of them becomes constrained, the entire system begins to compress around that limitation. Output no longer reflects total potential. It reflects the narrowest point through which the process must pass.

Cysteine defines the entry point into synthesis, setting the upper limit on how much new glutathione can be produced. When cysteine supply is sufficient, the first step proceeds and allows the system to respond to increased demand. When it is limited, the pathway cannot initiate at the required rate, and synthesis remains constrained regardless of glycine availability or enzyme activity. This creates a structural bottleneck where the system cannot expand its pool even when depletion signals are present.

Glycine defines completion of synthesis once the pathway has started. If glycine is diverted into competing pathways such as collagen production, nucleotide synthesis, or one-carbon metabolism, the intermediate formed in the first step cannot be converted into functional glutathione at the necessary rate. This creates a throughput limitation where the system initiates production but fails to deliver finished molecules in proportion to demand. The pathway remains active, but output is reduced.

Enzymatic capacity determines how quickly substrates can be converted into glutathione. Glutamate-cysteine ligase and glutathione synthetase must operate at rates that match substrate availability and cellular demand. Feedback inhibition, enzyme expression levels, and cofactor availability all influence this capacity. If enzyme activity is insufficient, substrates may be present but cannot be processed efficiently, creating a delay between availability and functional output.

Energy supply imposes a parallel constraint. Both steps of glutathione synthesis require ATP, linking production directly to the energetic state of the cell. When ATP levels are stable, synthesis can scale with demand. When energy is limited, the pathway slows, and production cannot increase even if substrates and enzymes are available. This creates a condition where the system is structurally capable of expansion but is held back by insufficient energy input.

NADPH availability controls the recovery side of the system. Recycling oxidized glutathione requires a continuous supply of reducing equivalents. When NADPH production matches demand, recycling maintains a high proportion of reduced glutathione. When it is limited, oxidized forms accumulate, and functional capacity declines even if total glutathione remains unchanged. This shifts the system toward depletion without necessarily reducing total concentration.

Transport and compartmental distribution introduce additional points of constraint. Glutathione synthesized in the cytosol must be delivered to compartments such as mitochondria, where local demand is high and direct synthesis does not occur. If transport mechanisms are insufficient or delayed, localized depletion can occur even when overall cellular levels appear adequate. Each compartment operates with its own balance of supply and demand, and bottlenecks at this level can produce region-specific instability.

Detoxification pathways can also act as bottlenecks by diverting glutathione out of the recycling cycle. Conjugation reactions bind glutathione to reactive compounds and export the resulting complexes from the cell. This removes glutathione from immediate use and requires additional synthesis to replace it. When conjugation rates increase, the system must compensate by increasing production. If it cannot, total available glutathione declines.

These bottlenecks do not operate independently. They interact and amplify one another. Limited cysteine reduces synthesis, which increases reliance on recycling. If NADPH is also limited, recycling cannot compensate, and the system shifts toward oxidation. Increased detoxification further removes glutathione from the pool, increasing demand for synthesis that cannot be met. The result is a compounded reduction in buffering capacity that emerges from the interaction of multiple constraints rather than a single failure point.

Glutathione function therefore reflects the integrity of the entire system rather than the presence of any one component. Bottlenecks define the operational limits of that system, determining how much reactive load can be processed, how quickly balance can be restored, and how stable the internal environment remains under changing conditions.

Substrate Limitation

Glutathione production depends on a continuous supply of specific amino acids, and limitation at this level constrains the entire system before enzymatic or energetic factors become relevant. The pathway requires glutamate, cysteine, and glycine, but these substrates are not equally available or equally prioritized within cellular metabolism. When supply falls short for any one of them, synthesis cannot proceed at the rate required to maintain or expand the glutathione pool, regardless of how active the enzymes are or how strong the demand signal becomes.

Cysteine imposes the most immediate constraint because it is maintained at low concentrations and must be generated or imported in real time. If cysteine availability drops, the first step of synthesis slows or stops, preventing formation of the intermediate structure that precedes glutathione. Glycine introduces a different form of limitation at the completion stage. It is broadly available but distributed across many pathways, and when demand in those pathways increases, less glycine is available to finalize glutathione construction. The result is a partial activation of the pathway where intermediates accumulate but finished output declines.

Substrate limitation is not only a matter of total intake but of allocation and timing. Amino acids are continuously routed into protein synthesis, structural maintenance, signaling molecules, and energy metabolism. Glutathione synthesis draws from the same pool and must compete with these processes. When overall demand increases, such as during tissue repair or rapid turnover, available substrates are redistributed, and glutathione production can become secondary even when buffering capacity is needed. This creates a mismatch between demand for redox control and the availability of materials required to support it.

Transport and intracellular distribution further influence substrate availability. Amino acids must be delivered into the cell and directed toward the cytosolic environment where synthesis occurs. Delays or inefficiencies in transport reduce the effective concentration of substrates at the site of assembly. Even when systemic levels appear adequate, localized shortages can limit production within specific cells or compartments.

The system responds to substrate limitation by increasing reliance on recycling existing glutathione, but this compensation has limits. Recycling preserves function temporarily, but it does not expand the total pool. If consumption continues at a rate that exceeds both recycling and limited synthesis, reduced glutathione declines and buffering capacity contracts. Over time, this leads to a sustained reduction in the system's ability to maintain redox balance.

Substrate limitation therefore defines the material boundary of glutathione production. It determines whether the system has the physical components required to build and maintain its buffering capacity. When substrates are sufficient and properly allocated, synthesis supports continuous adaptation to demand. When they are constrained, the system operates below its potential, and functional capacity declines despite intact enzymatic and energetic infrastructure.

Enzyme Inefficiency

Glutathione production and recovery depend on a small set of enzymes that must convert substrates at a rate that matches ongoing demand. When these enzymes operate below capacity, the system slows even if substrates and energy are available. The pathway remains intact, but throughput declines, creating a gap between what the system could produce and what it actually delivers into the glutathione pool.

The first point of sensitivity appears at glutamate-cysteine ligase, which controls entry into synthesis. This enzyme must align cysteine availability with ATP input to form the gamma-linked intermediate. If its activity is reduced, substrates accumulate without being converted, and initiation of synthesis becomes delayed or inconsistent. Feedback inhibition further shapes its behavior. When glutathione levels are high, the enzyme reduces its activity. When levels fall, that inhibition is relieved. If the enzyme cannot respond effectively to these signals, the system loses its ability to adjust production in proportion to demand.

The second step, carried out by glutathione synthetase, determines whether intermediate structures are converted into functional molecules. Reduced activity at this stage creates a buildup of partially assembled components that do not contribute to buffering capacity. The pathway appears active, but output remains low because completion is constrained. This type of inefficiency reduces effective production without altering substrate supply.

Recycling introduces another layer of dependence on enzyme performance. Glutathione reductase must convert oxidized glutathione back into its reduced form at a rate that matches consumption. If its activity is limited, oxidized glutathione accumulates even when NADPH is available. This shifts the balance of the pool toward forms that cannot participate in electron transfer, reducing functional capacity without necessarily reducing total concentration.

Enzyme inefficiency often reflects limitations in cofactors, structural integrity, or regulatory signaling rather than absence of the enzyme itself. These proteins require specific conditions to maintain their active configuration and catalytic rate. When those conditions are not met, reaction speed declines. Substrates remain present, but conversion slows, creating a bottleneck that reduces overall system performance.

The effects of inefficiency are cumulative. Reduced activity at one step increases pressure on other parts of the system. Slower synthesis increases reliance on recycling. If recycling is also limited, the system shifts toward depletion more rapidly. Delayed conversion at any stage extends the time reactive intermediates remain uncontained, increasing the likelihood of interaction with structural components.

Enzyme efficiency therefore defines how effectively the glutathione system translates available resources into functional output. It determines whether substrates are converted into active molecules at the rate required to maintain balance, and whether oxidized glutathione is restored quickly enough to sustain continuous reuse. When enzyme activity is aligned with demand, the system operates smoothly. When it is not, the pathway remains present but underperforms, and buffering capacity declines as a result.

Oxidative Overload

Oxidative overload occurs when the rate of reactive intermediate generation exceeds the combined capacity of glutathione to neutralize, recycle, and replace itself. Under normal conditions, reactive species are produced continuously as a byproduct of metabolism, particularly within the mitochondria during electron transport. These intermediates are intercepted by glutathione and related systems in real time, preventing them from interacting with structural components. When production increases beyond what the system can immediately contain, the balance shifts from controlled handling to accumulation.

The first effect of overload is accelerated oxidation of glutathione. As more reactive intermediates are present, more glutathione molecules are converted into their oxidized form. If recycling through glutathione reductase and NADPH supply can keep pace, the system maintains stability despite the increased demand. When it cannot, oxidized glutathione begins to accumulate and the proportion of reduced, functional molecules declines. This reduces the number of available thiol groups that can participate in further reactions, limiting the system's ability to intercept new reactive species.

Mitochondria are a primary site where this imbalance develops because they generate reactive intermediates as part of energy production. When electron flow through the transport chain becomes inefficient or overloaded, leakage increases and more reactive species are formed. Glutathione within the mitochondrial matrix must contain this output locally. If mitochondrial glutathione is depleted or not recycled efficiently, reactive intermediates begin to interact with mitochondrial membranes, proteins, and DNA, disrupting energy production and increasing further reactive generation in a feedback loop.

Oxidative overload also increases the rate at which glutathione is diverted into detoxification pathways. Reactive compounds and electrophiles bind to glutathione and are exported from the cell, removing those molecules from immediate reuse. This places additional demand on synthesis to replace the lost pool. If substrate availability or enzymatic capacity cannot support this increased need, total glutathione levels begin to decline alongside the shift toward oxidation.

As overload persists, the system transitions from rapid containment to delayed response. Reactive intermediates remain active for longer periods, increasing the likelihood of interaction with lipids, proteins, and nucleic acids. Lipid peroxidation accelerates, altering membrane structure. Protein oxidation affects enzyme function and signaling pathways. DNA damage increases the need for repair processes, further drawing on cellular resources.

Oxidative overload therefore reflects a failure of alignment between production, neutralization, and recovery. It is not defined solely by the presence of reactive species but by the inability of the glutathione system to maintain control over them. When buffering capacity is sufficient, increased production is absorbed without structural impact. When it is not, the system shifts toward accumulation, and reactive intermediates begin to alter the physical and functional integrity of the cell.

Genetics

Genetic variation shapes the baseline capacity of the glutathione system by determining how efficiently its components are built, regulated, and maintained. The enzymes that drive synthesis and recycling are encoded in the genome, and differences in these sequences influence how much enzyme is produced, how stable it is, and how effectively it performs under changing conditions. This establishes a starting architecture that defines how much glutathione can be generated, how quickly it can be restored, and how the system responds when demand increases.

Variation in the genes that control glutamate-cysteine ligase and glutathione synthetase directly affects synthesis throughput. Reduced expression or altered enzyme structure lowers the rate at which substrates are converted into glutathione, limiting how quickly the pool can expand when depletion signals are present. Even when cysteine and glycine are available, production remains capped by enzymatic capacity. This creates a fixed ceiling that cannot be overcome through substrate availability alone.

Recycling capacity is shaped by genetic control of glutathione reductase and the pathways that generate NADPH. If enzyme activity is reduced or NADPH production is constrained, oxidized glutathione accumulates more readily and recovery slows. The system shifts toward a higher proportion of inactive glutathione, reducing functional capacity without necessarily changing total concentration. This increases reliance on synthesis to maintain balance, placing additional pressure on substrate supply and enzymatic throughput.

Detoxification pathways introduce another layer of genetic influence. Enzymes responsible for conjugating glutathione to reactive compounds determine how quickly glutathione is removed from the active pool. Higher activity in these pathways increases clearance of reactive intermediates but also accelerates turnover of glutathione itself. If synthesis and recycling cannot match this increased demand, total available glutathione declines over time.

Transport systems that distribute glutathione and its substrates across compartments are also genetically defined. Variations in these systems influence how effectively glutathione reaches areas of high demand, particularly within mitochondria where local protection is critical. Reduced transport efficiency creates localized depletion even when overall cellular levels appear adequate, altering how different regions of the cell respond to reactive load.

These genetic constraints establish the operating range of the system, but they also create scenarios where baseline capacity is insufficient to meet modern levels of demand. When enzymatic throughput is reduced, recycling is slower, or substrate conversion pathways are less efficient, the system cannot maintain optimal glutathione levels through normal metabolic input alone. In these cases, additional support becomes necessary to compensate for structural limitations.

Supplementation becomes relevant at this point because it can increase substrate availability, support rate-limiting steps, or provide glutathione in forms that bypass parts of thc synthesis pathway. This does not override genetic architecture, but it can raise the functional output within those constraints. For individuals with reduced synthesis or recycling capacity, this added input can help restore the balance between consumption and recovery, allowing the system to maintain a higher proportion of active glutathione under sustained demand.

Genetics therefore defines both the limits and the requirements of the glutathione system. It determines how efficiently the system operates under baseline conditions and whether additional support is required to maintain stability when reactive load increases. The outcome is not determined by genetics alone, but by how those genetic constraints interact with substrate supply, energy availability, and external stressors that continuously shape demand.

PART VI

DEFICIENCY PATTERNS

What happens when the system can't keep up

Chapter 16

Early Depletion

Early depletion begins before total glutathione levels fall to visibly low ranges. The shift starts at the level of functional balance, where the proportion of reduced glutathione declines relative to the oxidized form. The total pool may still appear adequate, but its ability to participate in redox reactions is already compromised. This stage reflects a mismatch between consumption and recovery, where reactive load increases or recycling slows just enough to alter the internal ratio without immediately collapsing the system.

The first change occurs in the speed of recycling. Glutathione continues to be oxidized as it neutralizes reactive intermediates, but the rate at which it is restored begins to lag. NADPH supply may be slightly constrained, or enzymatic efficiency may not fully scale with demand. As a result, oxidized glutathione accumulates in small but meaningful amounts, reducing the availability of active thiol groups. This does not stop redox control, but it slows response time and reduces buffering precision.

At the same time, synthesis may continue at baseline levels without increasing to match rising demand. Substrate availability, particularly cysteine and glycine, may be sufficient for maintenance but not for expansion. The system is still producing glutathione, but not at a rate that compensates for increased turnover. This creates a gradual contraction in effective capacity, where the system relies more heavily on recycling to maintain function.

Early depletion also alters how glutathione is distributed across compartments. Regions with higher demand, such as mitochondria, begin to experience localized strain first. Mitochondrial glutathione is consumed rapidly during energy production, and if import or local recycling does not keep pace, internal levels begin to decline. This leads to increased interaction between reactive intermediates and mitochondrial structures, subtly reducing efficiency of energy production and increasing further reactive output.

Detoxification pathways contribute to early depletion by removing glutathione from the immediate pool. Increased exposure to reactive compounds leads to higher rates of conjugation and export, which reduces the amount available for redox buffering. Even if recycling remains active, this diversion reduces the effective pool size and increases reliance on synthesis to replace what has been lost.

The system compensates during this stage by prioritizing essential functions. Glutathione is directed toward areas of highest need, and less critical processes receive reduced support. This redistribution maintains core cellular operations but reduces overall flexibility. The system can still respond to changes, but with less margin for error and slower recovery when additional stress is introduced.

Early depletion therefore represents a loss of reserve rather than a complete failure. The system remains functional but operates closer to its limits. Small increases in reactive load or further reductions in substrate availability can push it into a more pronounced state of imbalance. The transition is gradual, defined by declining efficiency and reduced capacity rather than immediate collapse, but it establishes the conditions under which more significant depletion can occur if underlying constraints are not resolved.

Loss of Buffering Capacity

Loss of buffering capacity begins when the glutathione system can no longer maintain a high proportion of molecules in the reduced, active state. The total amount of glutathione may still be present, but its functional availability declines as more of the pool remains oxidized or diverted into conjugated forms. This shift changes how the system behaves. Instead of intercepting reactive intermediates as they are generated, the response becomes delayed, allowing those intermediates to persist long enough to interact with cellular structures.

The underlying cause is a breakdown in the alignment between oxidation, reduction, and replacement. Reactive production continues at a steady or increased rate, pushing glutathione into its oxidized form. Recycling through glutathione reductase slows when NADPH supply cannot keep pace, and synthesis fails to expand the pool due to substrate limitation or enzymatic constraints. Each component of the system is still present, but they no longer operate in synchrony. The result is a progressive reduction in the number of active thiol groups available at any given moment.

As buffering capacity declines, reactive intermediates begin to accumulate between cycles of neutralization. This increases the probability of interaction with lipids, proteins, and nucleic acids. Lipid peroxidation alters membrane structure, reducing fluidity and disrupting signaling pathways that depend on membrane integrity. Protein oxidation changes enzyme conformation and slows reaction rates across multiple pathways. DNA becomes more susceptible to damage, increasing the need for repair processes that further draw on cellular resources.

Mitochondria are affected early because they generate reactive intermediates continuously as part of energy production. Reduced buffering capacity allows these intermediates to interfere with components of the electron transport system, lowering efficiency and increasing leakage. This creates a feedback loop where reduced energy output limits ATP and NADPH production, further impairing both synthesis and recycling of glutathione. The system becomes progressively less able to restore its own balance.

Loss of buffering capacity also shifts how the cell allocates glutathione. More of the available pool is directed toward immediate containment of reactive species and detoxification, leaving less available for maintenance of structural integrity and signaling control. This redistribution preserves short-term survival but reduces long-term stability, as underlying damage begins to accumulate in areas that receive less support.

The transition is not defined by a single threshold but by a change in system behavior. When buffering capacity is intact, reactive intermediates are contained quickly and do not persist. When it declines, containment becomes incomplete, and reactive species remain active long enough to alter cellular components. This marks the point where the glutathione system shifts from maintaining stability to managing ongoing disruption, reflecting a reduction in its ability to sustain internal conditions under continuous metabolic demand.

Slower Recovery

Slower recovery emerges when the system can no longer return oxidized glutathione to its reduced state at the same rate it is being consumed. Under stable conditions, recovery is rapid and continuous. Glutathione cycles through oxidation and reduction without accumulating in its inactive form, and the pool remains largely available for immediate use. When recovery slows, this cycle stretches out in time. Oxidized glutathione remains in that state longer, and the interval between use and restoration increases.

The first constraint appears at the level of reducing power. NADPH must supply electrons for glutathione reductase to reverse oxidation, and when its production does not match demand, the reduction step becomes rate-limited. Even if glutathione reductase is present and functional, it cannot operate at full capacity without a steady supply of NADPH. This creates a delay in restoring active glutathione, reducing the number of molecules available to respond to new reactive intermediates.

Synthesis cannot immediately compensate for this delay. Building new glutathione requires cysteine, glycine, enzyme activity, and ATP. This process operates on a longer timescale than recycling. When recovery slows, the system becomes increasingly dependent on synthesis to rebuild its pool, but synthesis cannot match the speed required to maintain rapid buffering. The result is a gap between consumption and restoration that persists across cycles.

Compartmental dynamics amplify this effect. Mitochondria, which rely on a stable internal pool of glutathione, experience reduced recovery directly when local NADPH supply is constrained. Because mitochondrial glutathione cannot be replenished instantly from the cytosol, delays in local recycling lead to a sustained reduction in available buffering capacity within that compartment. This affects electron transport efficiency and increases reactive output, further increasing demand on a system that is already recovering more slowly.

Detoxification pathways contribute by removing glutathione from the immediate cycle. When glutathione is conjugated and exported, it is no longer available for rapid recovery. The system must replace these molecules through synthesis, which further increases the time required to restore the pool. As this diversion continues, the proportion of glutathione engaged in immediate buffering declines.

Slower recovery changes the timing of the system rather than its structure. The same components remain in place, but they operate with reduced speed. Reactive intermediates persist longer between cycles of neutralization, increasing the likelihood of interaction with cellular structures. The system can still respond, but it does so with a delay that reduces precision and increases cumulative impact over time.

This shift marks a transition from rapid containment to lagged response. When recovery is efficient, the system maintains a tight control over reactive processes. When it slows, that control becomes intermittent, and the internal environment begins to reflect the presence of reactive intermediates for longer periods. The result is a gradual decline in stability driven not by complete failure, but by reduced speed in restoring functional capacity.

Chapter 17

Functional Breakdown

Functional breakdown occurs when the glutathione system can no longer maintain continuity between neutralization, recovery, and replacement. At this stage, the system is not simply strained or operating at reduced efficiency. It begins to lose coordination across its components. Oxidation proceeds faster than reduction, synthesis cannot rebuild the pool at a sufficient rate, and detoxification removes glutathione faster than it can be replaced. The result is a persistent deficit in functional glutathione, where the system no longer maintains control over reactive processes in real time.

The defining feature of this stage is the collapse of the reduced to oxidized balance. Glutathione remains present, but a larger proportion exists in forms that cannot participate in electron transfer. Recycling is no longer able to restore oxidized glutathione at the rate required to sustain buffering, and NADPH supply becomes a limiting factor in maintaining recovery. As this imbalance persists, the system transitions from a dynamic cycle into a state where oxidation accumulates faster than it can be resolved.

Mitochondrial function becomes progressively unstable under these conditions. As reactive intermediates are no longer contained effectively, they begin to interfere with components of the electron transport system. This reduces efficiency of energy production and increases electron leakage, which in turn generates additional reactive species. The system enters a feedback loop where reduced energy output limits ATP and NADPH availability, further impairing both synthesis and recycling of glutathione. Each cycle reinforces the imbalance rather than correcting it.

Membrane integrity begins to degrade as lipid peroxidation accelerates. Phospholipids that form the structural basis of cellular membranes are altered by reactive interactions, changing membrane fluidity and permeability. This disrupts signaling pathways that depend on membrane organization and affects transport processes that regulate movement of substrates and ions. As membrane structure becomes less stable, the cell loses its ability to maintain controlled internal conditions.

Protein function declines as oxidative modifications alter enzyme structure and activity. Catalytic sites become less efficient, signaling pathways lose precision, and structural proteins begin to accumulate damage. These changes reduce the effectiveness of processes that depend on coordinated enzyme activity, including those required for repair and recovery. The system becomes less capable of correcting its own imbalance as the proteins responsible for those corrections lose functionality.

DNA integrity is increasingly challenged as reactive intermediates persist longer within the cell. Damage accumulates at a rate that exceeds repair capacity, placing additional strain on systems that rely on nucleotide availability and energy input. Repair processes continue to operate, but they compete with other demands for limited resources, reducing their overall effectiveness.

Detoxification pathways remain active but contribute to depletion by continuously removing glutathione from the system. As reactive compounds are conjugated and exported, the requirement for new synthesis increases. When synthesis cannot match this demand, total glutathione levels decline alongside functional capacity, further reducing the system's ability to respond.

Functional breakdown therefore represents a shift from controlled processing to unmanaged accumulation. The system retains its components, but they no longer operate in a coordinated manner that maintains stability. Reactive intermediates persist, structural components are progressively altered, and recovery mechanisms cannot restore balance at the required rate. The outcome is a state where the internal environment reflects ongoing disruption rather than controlled regulation, driven by the loss of alignment across the processes that sustain glutathione function.

Detox Slowdown

Detox slowdown begins when the rate at which reactive compounds are processed and cleared falls below the rate at which they are generated or introduced. Glutathione sits at the center of this system, acting as the primary molecule that binds and prepares these compounds for removal. When glutathione availability declines in its reduced, functional form, the conjugation process slows. Reactive intermediates remain unbound for longer periods, increasing the probability that they will interact with cellular structures instead of being directed into clearance pathways.

The slowdown is not caused by a single failure but by a reduction in coordinated throughput across multiple steps. Phase I reactions continue to modify compounds, often increasing their reactivity as part of the conversion process. These intermediates are then expected to be rapidly neutralized through glutathione conjugation in Phase II. When glutathione is limited or recycling is delayed, this second step cannot keep pace. The system begins to accumulate partially processed compounds that are more reactive than their original forms, increasing internal chemical stress rather than resolving it.

Glutathione conjugation requires both sufficient substrate and active enzyme systems to attach glutathione to these intermediates. When the available pool of reduced glutathione declines, fewer molecules are available to participate in these reactions. Even if enzymes are present and functional, the reaction rate drops because the substrate is not available at the required concentration. This creates a bottleneck where detoxification capacity is defined by glutathione availability rather than enzyme presence.

Export mechanisms also contribute to the slowdown. Once glutathione conjugates are formed, they must be transported out of the cell for further processing and elimination. If transport capacity is reduced or overwhelmed, conjugates accumulate within the cell, tying up glutathione in forms that are no longer available for immediate use. This reduces the effective pool of glutathione even further, compounding the limitation at the level of conjugation.

Energy and reducing equivalents influence detox throughput as well. ATP is required for transport processes, and NADPH supports the recycling of glutathione that sustains ongoing conjugation. When these inputs are limited, both the formation and clearance of conjugates slow, extending the time reactive intermediates remain active within the system.

As detox slows, the system shifts from rapid clearance to partial processing. Reactive compounds persist longer, interact more frequently with membranes, proteins, and DNA, and generate additional reactive intermediates through secondary reactions. This increases the overall load that the glutathione system must handle at a time when its capacity is already reduced.

Detox slowdown therefore reflects a reduction in flow through the entire clearance architecture. It is defined by delayed conjugation, constrained transport, and reduced recycling, all of which extend the presence of reactive compounds within the cell. The result is an accumulation of intermediates that the system can no longer process efficiently, marking a transition from controlled elimination to sustained internal exposure.

Incomplete Inflammatory Cycles

Inflammation is designed to move through a defined sequence that begins with activation and ends with resolution. The initial phase increases reactive production, recruits immune cells, and alters local metabolism to contain damage or remove a threat. The resolution phase then reverses these changes, clears residual intermediates, and restores structural stability. Glutathione is required at both ends of this process. It supports controlled generation of reactive species during activation and is then used to shut that activity down by neutralizing excess intermediates and restoring redox balance. When glutathione capacity is reduced, the system can initiate inflammation but cannot complete it.

The breakdown appears at the transition point between activation and resolution. Reactive intermediates that were produced to carry out immune functions remain present because they are not neutralized efficiently. This prolongs signaling pathways that depend on oxidative input, keeping immune cells in an activated state beyond their intended timeframe. Instead of a contained response followed by shutdown, the system remains partially engaged, maintaining a low level of activity that continues to generate reactive output.

Glutathione is also required to restore the chemical environment that allows resolution signals to take effect. Many of the processes that terminate inflammation depend on shifting the intracellular environment back toward a reduced state. When glutathione is insufficient, this shift does not occur fully. Resolution signals are generated but cannot execute effectively because the surrounding conditions still favor activation. The system remains in a state where initiation signals and termination signals are present at the same time, but neither fully dominates.

This incomplete cycling increases overall demand on the glutathione system. Ongoing low-level activation continues to produce reactive intermediates, which further consume the limited glutathione pool. At the same time, detoxification pathways remain active, removing glutathione through conjugation and export. The system is therefore placed under continuous pressure without a defined endpoint, accelerating depletion while preventing recovery.

Mitochondria contribute to this state by increasing reactive output during sustained activation. As energy demand rises in immune cells, electron transport activity increases, generating additional reactive intermediates that must be contained locally. When mitochondrial glutathione is insufficient, this output is not controlled effectively, reinforcing the activated state and further delaying resolution.

The structural impact of incomplete cycles accumulates over time. Persistent reactive intermediates alter membrane composition, disrupt signaling precision, and modify protein function. These changes feed back into the inflammatory system, making activation more likely and resolution more difficult with each cycle. The system becomes biased toward continued activity rather than completion.

Incomplete inflammatory cycles therefore reflect a failure to close the loop of activation and resolution. The system initiates a response but cannot restore the conditions required to end it. Glutathione depletion sits at the center of this failure, limiting the ability to neutralize residual intermediates and reestablish the reduced environment necessary for resolution. The result is a sustained, low-level inflammatory state that persists not because activation is excessive, but because completion is incomplete.

Chapter 18

System Instability

System instability emerges when the glutathione network loses its ability to maintain consistent control over redox conditions across time and compartments. Earlier stages reflect reduced capacity or slower recovery, but the system still behaves predictably. In this stage, behavior becomes variable. The system alternates between partial control and loss of control depending on moment-to-moment demand, substrate availability, and energy state. Stability is replaced by fluctuation, where short periods of adequate buffering are followed by periods of accumulation and delayed response.

The core issue is loss of synchronization. Oxidation, reduction, synthesis, and detoxification no longer operate in coordinated alignment. At times, recycling may temporarily restore a portion of the glutathione pool, creating a short window of improved function. As demand continues or increases, that restored capacity is consumed faster than it can be replaced, and the system shifts back toward oxidation. These oscillations occur because each component of the system responds at a different rate and with different constraints, producing uneven output rather than a steady state.

NADPH supply becomes inconsistent under these conditions, contributing to variability in recovery. Periods of adequate reducing power allow glutathione reductase to restore oxidized glutathione efficiently, but when NADPH production drops, recovery slows and oxidized forms accumulate. This creates alternating phases of higher and lower functional glutathione availability, which directly affects how well reactive intermediates are contained.

Substrate availability also fluctuates, particularly for cysteine and glycine. Changes in dietary input, metabolic demand, and allocation across competing pathways alter how much substrate is available for synthesis at any given time. When substrate levels rise, synthesis increases and temporarily supports recovery. When they fall, production declines and the system becomes more reliant on recycling, which may already be constrained. This variability feeds into the overall instability of the system.

Mitochondrial behavior amplifies these fluctuations. As energy production becomes less efficient, reactive output becomes less predictable. Periods of higher electron leakage increase demand on glutathione, accelerating consumption. When mitochondrial function stabilizes briefly, reactive output decreases, allowing partial recovery. These shifts contribute to an oscillating pattern where demand and capacity are rarely aligned.

Detoxification pathways continue to remove glutathione from the system, but the rate of removal may not match the variable rate of replacement. During periods of higher exposure or increased conjugation activity, glutathione is depleted more rapidly. If synthesis and recycling cannot compensate during these intervals, the system enters a lower capacity state that persists until inputs improve.

System instability therefore reflects a loss of steady-state control. The glutathione system no longer maintains a consistent buffer against reactive processes but instead moves between partial containment and partial overload. This variability increases the likelihood of structural interactions during periods of low capacity and reduces the system's ability to maintain stable internal conditions over time.

Increased Oxidative Damage

Increased oxidative damage appears when reactive intermediates remain active long enough to interact with structural components before they are neutralized. Under stable conditions, glutathione intercepts these intermediates as they are formed, limiting their movement and preventing contact with membranes, proteins, and nucleic acids. When buffering capacity declines or recovery slows, this interception becomes incomplete. Reactive species persist between cycles of neutralization, increasing the probability of direct interaction with cellular structures.

Membranes are affected first because they present a large surface area of reactive lipids. Polyunsaturated fatty acids within phospholipids are particularly susceptible to chain reactions that propagate once initiated. When glutathione and associated systems cannot terminate these reactions quickly, lipid peroxidation spreads across the membrane, altering fluidity and permeability. This changes how receptors function, how signals are transmitted, and how ions and substrates move across the membrane. The structural integrity of the membrane shifts from controlled organization to a more disordered state.

Proteins undergo modification as reactive intermediates interact with amino acid side chains that are sensitive to oxidation. Enzymes lose efficiency as their active sites are altered, reducing reaction rates across multiple pathways. Structural proteins accumulate damage that affects cellular architecture, and signaling proteins transmit distorted information as their conformation changes. These effects do not occur in isolation. Reduced enzyme performance feeds back into the system by slowing processes required for repair and recovery.

DNA becomes increasingly exposed as buffering declines. Reactive intermediates that are not neutralized can interact with nucleotides, creating lesions that require repair. As damage accumulates, repair systems draw on energy and substrate resources that are already limited. This increases the burden on the system and diverts capacity away from other processes, including glutathione synthesis and recycling.

Mitochondria amplify this progression. As oxidative damage affects components of the electron transport system, efficiency declines and electron leakage increases. This generates additional reactive intermediates, further increasing demand on a system that is already operating below capacity. The cycle reinforces itself, with damage increasing production and increased production accelerating damage.

The accumulation of oxidative damage reflects a shift in system behavior from containment to interaction. Reactive intermediates are no longer confined to controlled reactions but begin to alter the physical structure of the cell. Each interaction reduces functional capacity in the affected component, and the combined effect across membranes, proteins, and DNA produces a progressive decline in overall system performance.

Loss of Resolution Capacity

Loss of resolution capacity occurs when the system can still initiate responses but cannot complete them and return to baseline. The defining feature is not failure to react but failure to shut down and restore structure once the response has served its purpose. Glutathione is central to this transition because it resets the intracellular environment from an activated, reactive state back to a reduced, stable state. When that reset cannot occur fully, processes remain partially engaged and the system drifts into a prolonged intermediate condition.

Resolution requires removal of residual reactive intermediates that were generated during activation. These intermediates function as signals during the initial phase, but they must be cleared to terminate those signals. When glutathione availability is reduced or recycling is delayed, these intermediates persist. Signaling pathways that depend on oxidative input continue to operate, keeping transcriptional and enzymatic activity in a state of partial activation. The system no longer distinguishes clearly between active and resolved states.

This failure extends to lipid signaling as well. Membrane-derived signals that guide the resolution phase depend on a controlled redox environment to form and function correctly. When oxidative conditions persist, these signals are either not generated in the correct proportions or are altered before they can execute their function. The sequence that normally transitions inflammation toward resolution becomes fragmented, with initiation signals still present and termination signals unable to complete their effect.

Cellular cleanup processes also depend on sufficient glutathione to proceed efficiently. Damaged proteins and lipids must be processed and removed, and intracellular conditions must support the enzymatic systems responsible for this work. When glutathione is limited, these processes slow. Partially damaged components remain within the system longer, continuing to interfere with normal function and contributing to ongoing reactive production.

Mitochondria remain in a state of elevated activity under these conditions. As long as reactive intermediates are not fully neutralized, electron transport remains less efficient and continues to produce additional reactive output. This sustains the internal environment that favors activation over resolution, reinforcing the incomplete state.

Loss of resolution capacity therefore reflects a breakdown in the final stage of system control. The system can respond, but it cannot return to baseline. Reactive intermediates persist, signaling remains active, and structural repair is incomplete. This creates a continuous demand for glutathione without a corresponding reduction in load, preventing recovery and establishing a state where processes remain open instead of being fully completed.

PART VII

DISEASE AS LOSS OF COMPLETION

Unifying disease through glutathione failure

Chapter 19

Chronic Inflammation

Chronic inflammation develops when activation persists without completion and the system loses the ability to return to a stable baseline. The process is not driven by a single continuous trigger but by repeated cycles that fail to resolve. Each cycle begins with activation, produces reactive intermediates, and then stalls before resolution is complete. Glutathione sits at the center of this failure because it is required to terminate reactive signaling, restore redox balance, and allow the system to shut down. When glutathione capacity is insufficient, the system remains in a partially activated state that sustains itself over time.

The defining feature of this condition is persistence of signaling rather than intensity of response. Reactive intermediates remain present at levels that are lower than acute activation but high enough to maintain continuous stimulation of inflammatory pathways. These intermediates alter transcriptional activity, enzyme behavior, and cellular communication, keeping immune processes engaged even in the absence of a new initiating event. The system is no longer cycling cleanly between activation and resolution. It remains in an extended intermediate state where both processes are partially active.

Mitochondrial behavior reinforces this persistence. Reduced efficiency in electron transport increases leakage and generates a steady supply of reactive intermediates that sustain signaling. At the same time, reduced ATP and NADPH production limit both glutathione synthesis and recycling, preventing recovery of buffering capacity. This creates a self-reinforcing loop where ongoing reactive production maintains activation while limiting the system's ability to restore balance.

Membrane structure and signaling are altered as lipid peroxidation accumulates. Phospholipids that normally support organized receptor function become disordered, changing how signals are received and transmitted. This disrupts normal feedback mechanisms that would otherwise help terminate inflammatory signaling. The system becomes less responsive to signals that promote resolution and more sensitive to signals that sustain activation.

Protein function is progressively affected as oxidative modifications alter enzyme activity and signaling pathways. Enzymes involved in resolution become less efficient, while those involved in activation remain engaged due to persistent reactive input. This imbalance shifts the system toward continued activity rather than completion, even when external triggers are minimal.

Detoxification pathways remain active but operate within a constrained system. Glutathione is continuously used to process reactive compounds and exported through conjugation pathways, reducing the available pool for redox buffering. As this diversion continues, synthesis and recycling cannot fully replace what is lost, maintaining the system in a reduced capacity state that favors persistence of inflammation.

Chronic inflammation therefore reflects a system that has lost the ability to complete its own processes. Activation continues at a low but sustained level, resolution remains incomplete, and the internal environment supports ongoing reactive signaling. Glutathione depletion is not the sole cause but acts as a central limiting factor that prevents the system from restoring the conditions required to shut down inflammatory activity and return to stability.

Failure to Resolve Immune Activation

Failure to resolve immune activation begins when the system completes the initiation phase but cannot terminate it. Immune cells activate correctly, reactive intermediates are produced, and signaling pathways engage as expected, but the conditions required to shut these processes down do not reappear. Glutathione is required to restore the intracellular environment from an oxidative, activated state back to a reduced state that permits resolution. When this restoration does not occur, activation signals continue to propagate even after the original trigger has been handled.

The persistence of reactive intermediates is the primary driver of this failure. These molecules act as signaling inputs during activation, but they must be cleared to terminate those signals. When glutathione availability is reduced or recycling is delayed, reactive intermediates remain present and continue to stimulate transcription factors and enzymatic pathways that sustain immune activity. The system is not receiving new input, but it behaves as if activation is still required because the internal signals have not been reset.

Resolution requires a coordinated shift in signaling that depends on a controlled redox environment. As glutathione restores balance, signaling pathways that promote termination become dominant and immune cells transition out of their active state. When this shift is incomplete, resolution signals are generated but cannot execute effectively. Activation and resolution pathways operate at the same time, creating a condition where neither process fully completes. The system remains locked in a partial state of engagement.

Mitochondrial output contributes to this persistence. Continued production of reactive intermediates during energy generation reinforces the oxidative environment that sustains activation. Reduced efficiency in electron transport increases leakage, and without sufficient glutathione to contain it, this output maintains signaling that prevents shutdown. The cell remains in a state that favors activity over recovery.

Cellular cleanup processes are also impaired. Removal of damaged proteins, lipids, and other byproducts of activation requires a stable redox environment. When glutathione is limited, these processes slow, leaving residual material that continues to stimulate immune pathways. This extends the duration of activation beyond what is required and increases the likelihood of repeated cycles.

The system shifts from event-driven activation to state-driven activation. Instead of responding to discrete challenges and then resolving, it maintains a background level of activity that persists independently of new triggers. This state increases demand on glutathione continuously, preventing recovery and reinforcing the conditions that sustain activation.

Failure to resolve immune activation therefore reflects a breakdown in the final stage of the inflammatory sequence. The system initiates a response but cannot restore the conditions required to end it. Glutathione depletion limits the ability to clear reactive intermediates and reset signaling, leaving the immune system in a prolonged state of partial activation that becomes self-sustaining over time.

Chapter 20

Metabolic Disease

Metabolic disease emerges when energy production, redox control, and structural integrity lose coordination and begin to reinforce one another in a destabilized state. The system is no longer operating as a set of aligned processes that convert substrates into usable energy while maintaining internal balance. Instead, energy production generates reactive intermediates that are not fully contained, redox buffering cannot restore stability, and structural components begin to degrade. Glutathione sits at the center of this shift because it links energy metabolism to redox control and determines whether reactive output remains contained or begins to alter system behavior.

The initial disruption occurs at the level of mitochondrial function. As electron transport becomes less efficient, leakage increases and more reactive intermediates are generated during energy production. Under stable conditions, glutathione within the mitochondrial matrix intercepts these intermediates and prevents them from interacting with components of the transport system. When glutathione availability declines or recovery slows, these intermediates begin to interfere with electron flow itself. This reduces ATP output and increases further leakage, creating a feedback loop where reduced efficiency increases reactive production, and increased reactive production further reduces efficiency.

This shift alters how substrates are processed. Instead of being converted cleanly into energy, they are handled through pathways that generate more intermediate stress. Lipid oxidation becomes less controlled, producing partially processed intermediates that require additional detoxification. Glucose handling becomes less precise as signaling pathways that regulate uptake and storage are altered by oxidative modifications. The system begins to favor patterns of storage and incomplete utilization rather than efficient conversion and turnover.

Membrane structure plays a central role in this transition. Phospholipid composition determines how receptors, transporters, and signaling complexes function. As lipid peroxidation alters these membranes, signaling pathways that control metabolic decisions become less reliable. Insulin signaling is affected at the level of receptor function and downstream signaling cascades, reducing the cell's ability to respond appropriately to circulating nutrients. Transport of substrates into the cell becomes less controlled, and distribution within the cell becomes less organized.

Redox imbalance extends into regulatory systems that control metabolic pathways. Enzymes that depend on specific structural configurations lose efficiency as oxidative modifications accumulate. Pathways that require precise coordination between multiple enzymes begin to slow or fragment, leading to accumulation of intermediates that would normally be processed further. This increases the burden on detoxification systems and further consumes glutathione.

Detoxification demand rises as a result of these changes. Partially processed substrates and reactive byproducts must be conjugated and removed, increasing the rate at which glutathione is diverted out of the active pool. As this diversion continues, synthesis and recycling must increase to maintain levels. When they cannot, total glutathione availability declines alongside functional capacity, further reducing the system's ability to contain reactive output.

The system transitions from regulated metabolism to unstable processing. Energy production becomes less efficient, substrate handling becomes less precise, and reactive intermediates persist longer within the cellular environment. Each of these changes feeds into the others, creating a state where metabolic pathways no longer operate in a coordinated manner that maintains stability.

Metabolic disease therefore reflects a breakdown in the integration between energy production, redox buffering, and structural organization. Glutathione depletion is not the sole cause, but it removes the system's ability to contain reactive intermediates and restore balance, allowing disruptions in one area to propagate across the entire metabolic network.

Mitochondrial Inefficiency

Mitochondrial inefficiency develops when electron flow through the transport system loses precision and begins to leak before completing the full sequence of energy conversion. Under stable conditions, electrons move through a defined chain, driving proton gradients that produce ATP while minimizing release of reactive intermediates. Glutathione within the mitochondrial matrix contains the small amount of reactive output that is generated as part of this process. When glutathione availability declines or recovery slows, this containment becomes incomplete, and leaked electrons form reactive species that remain active within the matrix.

As these intermediates accumulate, they begin to interfere with the components that control electron flow. Protein complexes within the transport system lose efficiency as oxidative modifications alter their structure. This reduces the rate at which electrons are transferred, increasing the likelihood that additional electrons will escape prematurely. The system shifts from controlled flow to partial leakage, where energy conversion produces less ATP and more reactive byproducts at the same time.

Reduced ATP output feeds back into the system by limiting processes that require energy input, including glutathione synthesis and transport. As ATP availability declines, the ability to rebuild and distribute glutathione is reduced, further lowering buffering capacity within the mitochondria. This creates a reinforcing loop where decreased containment increases damage, and increased damage further decreases containment.

NADPH availability within the mitochondria also becomes constrained as inefficiency progresses. Local recycling of glutathione depends on a steady supply of reducing equivalents, and when mitochondrial metabolism becomes disorganized, NADPH production does not keep pace with demand. This slows the conversion of oxidized glutathione back into its reduced form, allowing oxidized species to accumulate and reducing the proportion of active molecules available for containment.

Membrane integrity within the mitochondria is affected as lipid peroxidation alters the composition of the inner membrane. This membrane is critical for maintaining the proton gradient that drives ATP production. Changes in its structure reduce the efficiency of gradient formation and increase proton leakage, further lowering ATP output and increasing the demand for electron transport activity. This increases reactive production in a system that is already struggling to contain it.

The net effect is a shift in mitochondrial behavior from efficient energy conversion to unstable processing. Substrates continue to enter the system, but they are not converted into energy with the same precision. Instead, they generate a combination of reduced ATP and increased reactive intermediates, both of which contribute to broader metabolic disruption.

Mitochondrial inefficiency therefore reflects a loss of alignment between electron flow, energy production, and redox control. Glutathione depletion removes the system's ability to contain reactive output at the point of generation, allowing small disruptions in electron transport to expand into sustained inefficiency that affects the entire metabolic network.

Energy Instability

Energy instability develops when ATP production no longer tracks consistently with demand and begins to fluctuate based on moment-to-moment changes in mitochondrial performance. Under stable conditions, substrate input, electron transport, and ATP generation operate as a coordinated system that delivers a steady output. Glutathione maintains this stability by containing reactive intermediates that would otherwise disrupt electron flow. When glutathione capacity declines, that containment becomes inconsistent, and energy production shifts from steady output to variable performance.

The first change appears as reduced efficiency in converting substrates into ATP. Electron transport becomes less precise, and a portion of incoming energy is diverted into reactive intermediates instead of being captured as usable energy. This lowers the amount of ATP produced per unit of substrate. The system compensates by increasing throughput, pushing more substrates through the pathway to maintain output. This compensation increases electron flow but also increases leakage, generating more reactive intermediates in a system that is already struggling to contain them.

As reactive intermediates accumulate, they interfere with components of the transport system, further reducing efficiency. This creates a feedback pattern where reduced output leads to increased demand, increased demand increases reactive production, and increased reactive production further reduces output. ATP levels begin to fluctuate rather than remain stable, creating periods of relative sufficiency followed by periods of deficit.

NADPH production is affected alongside ATP because both depend on coordinated metabolic flow. As instability increases, NADPH supply becomes inconsistent, reducing the system's ability to recycle glutathione. This further decreases buffering capacity, allowing reactive intermediates to persist longer and amplify disruption within the mitochondria. The system loses both its energy output and its ability to protect that output from internal interference.

Membrane structure contributes to this instability. Changes in mitochondrial membrane composition alter proton gradient formation and increase leakage across the membrane. This reduces the efficiency of ATP synthesis and forces the system to work harder to maintain energy levels. Increased workload further stresses the electron transport system, increasing the likelihood of additional reactive production.

Energy instability affects all processes that depend on consistent ATP availability. Synthesis of glutathione slows when ATP is limited, transport processes become less reliable, and repair mechanisms lose efficiency. The system begins to prioritize immediate survival over maintenance, directing available energy toward essential functions while delaying processes that restore long-term stability.

The result is a system that cannot maintain a steady internal state. Energy output rises and falls based on transient conditions rather than remaining aligned with demand. Each fluctuation feeds back into redox imbalance, reducing glutathione capacity and increasing reactive interference. Energy instability therefore reflects a loss of coordinated control between substrate processing, electron transport, and redox buffering, where the system can no longer produce consistent output without generating internal disruption.

Chapter 21

Neurological Dysfunction

Neurological dysfunction emerges when the glutathione system can no longer maintain a stable chemical environment within neural tissue, where signaling depends on precise timing, membrane integrity, and tightly controlled redox conditions. The nervous system operates with minimal tolerance for fluctuation. Small changes in membrane composition, ion gradients, or neurotransmitter balance alter how signals are generated and transmitted. When glutathione capacity declines, reactive intermediates begin to persist within this environment, and the system shifts from precise signaling to variable, distorted output.

Neurons are particularly sensitive because they rely on continuous energy production and maintain high concentrations of polyunsaturated lipids within their membranes. These lipids support flexibility and rapid signaling, but they are also highly susceptible to peroxidation. When glutathione is insufficient to contain reactive intermediates, lipid peroxidation alters membrane structure, changing how receptors and ion channels function. Signal transmission becomes less predictable as membrane properties shift away from their optimal configuration.

Mitochondrial inefficiency amplifies these effects within neurons. Energy demand remains high to support ion gradients and neurotransmitter cycling, but reduced efficiency in electron transport increases reactive output while lowering ATP production. This creates a mismatch where the cell requires more energy to maintain function but produces less usable output. Reactive intermediates generated during this process further disrupt mitochondrial components, reinforcing the cycle of inefficiency.

Neurotransmitter systems are affected as oxidative conditions alter both synthesis and degradation pathways. Enzymes responsible for producing and breaking down neurotransmitters depend on stable structural conditions to function correctly. When these conditions are disrupted, neurotransmitter levels fluctuate, and signaling becomes less controlled. This affects communication between neurons, altering network behavior rather than isolated signaling events.

Glial cells, which support neuronal function and regulate the surrounding environment, also depend on glutathione to maintain stability. When their buffering capacity declines, their ability to regulate extracellular conditions weakens. This allows reactive intermediates and inflammatory signals to persist within the neural environment, further affecting neuronal behavior and increasing overall system instability.

Detoxification within the nervous system is constrained compared to other tissues, making reliance on glutathione even more critical. Reactive compounds that are not neutralized quickly remain within the local environment, increasing the likelihood of interaction with neural structures. This places additional demand on an already limited system, accelerating the decline in functional capacity.

The cumulative effect is a shift from controlled neural signaling to disrupted network behavior. Signal transmission becomes inconsistent, energy supply becomes unreliable, and structural integrity of membranes and proteins declines. These changes do not occur as isolated failures but as interconnected disruptions that alter how the nervous system processes and responds to information.

Neurological dysfunction therefore reflects a breakdown in the conditions required for precise signaling. Glutathione depletion removes the system's ability to maintain a stable redox environment, allowing reactive intermediates to interfere with energy production, membrane structure, and neurotransmitter regulation. The result is a system that continues to operate but does so with reduced accuracy and stability, producing functional impairment that emerges from loss of internal control rather than absence of activity.

Brain Vulnerability to Oxidative Stress

The brain operates under conditions that make it inherently exposed to oxidative disruption. It consumes a large share of the body's energy while relying on continuous mitochondrial activity to maintain ion gradients and support rapid signaling. This high rate of electron transport produces a steady baseline of reactive intermediates that must be contained in real time. Unlike other tissues that can tolerate fluctuations or reduce activity under stress, neural tissue must maintain constant function. This creates a narrow operating range where even small increases in reactive load can alter system behavior.

Membrane composition increases this vulnerability. Neuronal membranes are enriched with polyunsaturated fatty acids that provide the flexibility required for synaptic signaling and receptor function. These same lipids are structurally susceptible to peroxidation. When reactive intermediates are not neutralized quickly, chain reactions spread across the membrane, altering its physical properties. This changes how ion channels open and close, how receptors respond to neurotransmitters, and how signals are transmitted across synapses. The effect is not limited to a single pathway but alters the underlying structure that all signaling depends on.

Glutathione acts as the primary buffer that protects this environment, but its availability in neural tissue is tightly constrained. Neurons depend heavily on surrounding support cells to maintain glutathione supply, and intracellular reserves are limited relative to demand. When glutathione levels decline or recycling slows, reactive intermediates persist longer within the neuronal environment. This increases the likelihood of interaction with membranes, proteins, and mitochondrial components at the point where signaling precision is required.

Mitochondrial sensitivity further amplifies this exposure. Neurons rely on stable ATP production to maintain electrical gradients, but mitochondrial inefficiency increases reactive output while reducing energy availability. This creates a condition where the system produces more reactive intermediates at the same time that its ability to contain them is reduced. As reactive intermediates interfere with mitochondrial components, efficiency declines further, increasing both energy instability and oxidative load.

Repair capacity within the brain is also limited compared to other tissues. Neurons are not replaced easily, and structural damage accumulates over time rather than being removed through turnover. When oxidative damage affects proteins, lipids, or DNA within neurons, the system must maintain function despite that damage. This places additional demand on glutathione to contain further disruption while existing damage remains present.

Detoxification pathways are less robust in neural tissue, increasing reliance on local buffering systems. Reactive compounds that would be processed more efficiently in other tissues persist longer in the neural environment, increasing exposure time. This places additional pressure on glutathione to maintain control over reactive processes without the same level of external support.

Brain vulnerability to oxidative stress therefore reflects the combination of high reactive production, structurally sensitive membranes, constrained buffering capacity, and limited repair options. Glutathione is required to maintain stability within this environment, and when its capacity declines, the system becomes exposed to disruptions that alter signaling, energy production, and structural integrity simultaneously.

Chapter 22

Toxic Burden and Accumulation

Toxic burden accumulates when the rate of exposure and internal generation of reactive compounds exceeds the system's capacity to process, neutralize, and remove them. This is not a single event but a gradual shift in balance where compounds that should move through the system are retained for longer periods and begin to interact with cellular structures. Glutathione defines the throughput of this system because it is required to bind, stabilize, and direct these compounds toward elimination. When glutathione availability declines or turnover slows, processing becomes incomplete and accumulation begins.

The process starts with increased demand on conjugation pathways. Reactive compounds, electrophiles, and byproducts of metabolism are modified to become more reactive in earlier processing steps and must then be neutralized through binding. Glutathione attaches to these intermediates, forming complexes that can be transported out of the cell. When the supply of reduced glutathione is sufficient, this process proceeds continuously and prevents buildup. When supply is limited, fewer intermediates are conjugated, and more remain in their reactive form within the cellular environment.

As conjugation slows, partially processed compounds accumulate. These intermediates often have higher reactivity than their original forms because they have been altered to increase solubility or reactivity for processing. Without sufficient glutathione to complete the sequence, they persist in a state that allows interaction with membranes, proteins, and DNA. This increases internal chemical stress and creates additional demand on the glutathione system.

Export capacity becomes a secondary constraint. Once glutathione conjugates are formed, they must be transported out of the cell. If transport systems are saturated or operating below capacity, conjugates remain inside the cell, effectively sequestering glutathione in forms that are no longer available for immediate buffering. This reduces the active pool and increases reliance on synthesis to replace what has been bound and retained.

Accumulation also reflects incomplete recovery of glutathione components. After export, conjugates are broken down and their constituent amino acids can be reused for synthesis. When this recovery process is inefficient or delayed, the system loses material that would otherwise support ongoing production. This reduces substrate availability over time, further constraining synthesis and reinforcing the accumulation cycle.

Mitochondrial and cytosolic environments both contribute to this burden. Reactive intermediates generated internally add to the load that must be processed, while external exposures introduce additional compounds that compete for the same detoxification pathways. When these inputs increase simultaneously, the system becomes saturated, and accumulation accelerates.

The result is a shift from continuous flow to partial retention. Compounds that should be processed and cleared instead remain within the system, interacting with structural components and generating additional reactive intermediates. This increases the overall demand on glutathione at a time when its availability is already constrained.

Toxic burden therefore reflects a reduction in processing capacity relative to input. It is defined by slowed conjugation, constrained export, and incomplete recovery, all of which extend the presence of reactive compounds within the system. As accumulation increases, the glutathione system is placed under continuous demand without sufficient capacity to restore balance, reinforcing the cycle of buildup and depletion.

Incomplete Detox → Recirculation

Incomplete detoxification shifts the system from one of directional flow to one of repeated internal exposure. Under normal conditions, reactive compounds are processed through a sequence that converts them into forms that can be bound, transported, and eliminated. Glutathione plays a central role by attaching to these intermediates and stabilizing them for export. When this sequence is interrupted before completion, compounds that have already been modified are not cleared. They remain within the system or are reintroduced after partial processing, creating a cycle where the same molecules pass through multiple times without being fully removed.

The first disruption occurs at the level of conjugation. Reactive intermediates generated during earlier processing steps require sufficient reduced glutathione to be neutralized and prepared for elimination. When glutathione availability is limited, a portion of these intermediates remains unbound. These partially processed compounds are more reactive than their original forms and persist within the cellular environment, increasing the likelihood of interaction with structural components.

Even when conjugation occurs, incomplete downstream handling can return these compounds to circulation. Glutathione conjugates must be transported out of the cell and further processed into forms that can be excreted. If transport is delayed or downstream processing is inefficient, these conjugates can be broken down and reabsorbed, releasing reactive components back into the system. This creates a loop where compounds are repeatedly processed but not eliminated, increasing cumulative exposure.

Recirculation increases the effective load on the glutathione system without requiring additional external input. Each pass through the cycle consumes glutathione, either through repeated conjugation or through attempts to neutralize reactive intermediates that persist after incomplete processing. This places continuous demand on synthesis and recycling, accelerating depletion even when exposure levels remain constant.

The presence of recirculating compounds also sustains reactive signaling within the system. As these intermediates move through tissues multiple times, they continue to interact with membranes, proteins, and signaling pathways, generating additional reactive intermediates and maintaining a state of ongoing chemical activity. This prolongs the conditions that drive glutathione consumption and delays recovery of buffering capacity.

Energy and transport capacity influence whether detoxification proceeds to completion or returns compounds to circulation. ATP-dependent transport systems must move conjugates out of the cell, and downstream pathways must convert them into excretable forms. When these processes are constrained, the system cannot maintain forward progression, and recirculation becomes more likely.

Incomplete detoxification therefore transforms a linear clearance process into a cyclical exposure pattern. Instead of reducing internal load with each pass, the system reintroduces partially processed compounds, increasing total demand on glutathione and extending the presence of reactive intermediates within the body. The result is a sustained burden that persists not because of new input, but because existing compounds are not fully removed from the system.

Chapter 23

Aging as Redox Failure

Aging emerges as a progressive loss of the system's ability to maintain redox completion across time. The defining feature is not simply the accumulation of damage, but the inability to continuously restore the internal environment after each cycle of metabolic activity. Every cycle of energy production, detoxification, and signaling generates reactive intermediates that must be contained and resolved. Glutathione enables that resolution by neutralizing these intermediates and returning the system to a reduced, stable state. As this capacity declines, each cycle leaves behind a small amount of unresolved change. Over time, these changes accumulate and alter the structure and behavior of the system.

The process begins with a gradual reduction in synthesis capacity. Substrate availability becomes less consistent, enzymatic throughput declines, and energy required for construction is not always sufficient to support expansion of the glutathione pool. At the same time, recycling efficiency decreases as NADPH production becomes less reliable. This reduces the speed at which oxidized glutathione is restored to its active form. The system shifts toward a state where consumption slightly exceeds recovery, creating a persistent imbalance that compounds over time.

Mitochondria play a central role in this transition. As efficiency declines, electron leakage increases and generates a higher baseline level of reactive intermediates. These intermediates are not fully contained when glutathione capacity is reduced, leading to progressive alteration of mitochondrial components. Reduced ATP output limits both synthesis and transport of glutathione, while reduced NADPH limits recycling. This creates a reinforcing loop where declining energy production and reduced buffering capacity amplify one another.

Membrane structure changes as lipid peroxidation accumulates. Phospholipid composition shifts, altering fluidity and disrupting the organization of signaling complexes embedded within the membrane. These changes affect how cells respond to external inputs and how internal signals are transmitted. Over time, the system loses the ability to coordinate responses with the same precision, leading to variability in function across tissues.

Protein integrity declines as oxidative modifications accumulate. Enzymes lose efficiency, structural proteins lose stability, and signaling pathways become less reliable. These changes reduce the system's ability to maintain its own processes, including those required for repair and recovery. Each cycle of damage and incomplete repair increases the burden on the system and reduces its capacity to respond to new demands.

DNA repair becomes less effective as damage accumulates and energy availability declines. Repair systems continue to operate but compete for resources with other processes that are also under strain. This leads to a gradual increase in unrepaired or misrepaired lesions, further altering cellular function and increasing variability across cells and tissues.

Detoxification capacity declines as glutathione is continuously consumed and not fully replaced. Reactive compounds remain within the system for longer periods, increasing cumulative exposure and contributing to further reactive production. This extends the burden across time, reinforcing the cycle of depletion and accumulation.

Aging therefore reflects a system that can no longer complete its own cycles. Each cycle leaves residual disruption because the processes required to restore balance are operating below capacity. Glutathione depletion is central to this shift because it removes the system's ability to resolve reactive intermediates and return to baseline. The result is a gradual transition from controlled, repeatable function to accumulated variability and structural change that defines the aging process as a failure of redox completion.

Damage Outpacing Repair

Damage begins to outpace repair when the rate at which reactive interactions alter cellular structures exceeds the system's ability to restore those structures to their original state. Under stable conditions, damage and repair operate in parallel. Reactive intermediates are generated, small amounts of structural alteration occur, and repair systems correct those changes before they accumulate. Glutathione maintains this balance by limiting the number of interactions that occur and by supporting the conditions required for repair processes to function efficiently. When glutathione capacity declines, this balance shifts, and repair can no longer keep pace with ongoing damage.

The first change appears as an increase in unrepaired modifications across membranes, proteins, and DNA. Reactive intermediates persist longer and interact more frequently with these structures, increasing the total number of events that require correction. Repair systems continue to operate, but they are limited by energy availability, substrate supply, and enzymatic efficiency. As demand increases, these systems become saturated, and a portion of damage remains uncorrected after each cycle.

Energy availability becomes a central constraint. Repair processes require ATP to operate, and mitochondrial inefficiency reduces the amount of usable energy produced. At the same time, NADPH is required to maintain the redox environment that supports repair enzymes and recycling systems. When both ATP and NADPH are limited, repair processes slow, extending the time required to resolve each event. This increases the overlap between new damage and incomplete repair from previous cycles.

Structural integrity begins to shift as unrepaired damage accumulates. Membrane composition changes as lipid peroxidation products are not fully replaced, altering fluidity and signaling behavior. Proteins with oxidative modifications remain in circulation longer, reducing the efficiency of pathways that depend on their function. DNA lesions persist, increasing the burden on replication and transcription processes.

These changes reduce the system's ability to maintain its own structure, making subsequent damage more likely and more difficult to repair.

Detoxification pathways contribute indirectly to this imbalance. As reactive compounds accumulate and require processing, glutathione is diverted into conjugation and export, reducing the pool available for redox buffering. This increases the likelihood of additional damage events while repair systems are already under strain. The system enters a state where both prevention and correction are operating below capacity.

The progression is cumulative rather than immediate. Each cycle leaves behind a small amount of unresolved damage, which alters the baseline from which the next cycle begins. Over time, these residual changes accumulate and begin to affect overall system behavior, reducing efficiency and increasing variability across processes.

Damage outpacing repair therefore reflects a loss of equilibrium between two continuous processes. It is defined by an increase in the number of damage events and a simultaneous decrease in the system's ability to resolve them. Glutathione depletion sits at the center of this shift by allowing more interactions to occur while reducing the conditions required for effective repair, leading to a gradual accumulation of structural and functional disruption.

PART VIII

RESTORATION ARCHITECTURE

How to rebuild the system instead of forcing outcomes

Chapter 24

Restoring Synthesis Capacity

Restoring synthesis capacity requires rebuilding the conditions that allow glutathione production to operate at a rate that matches or exceeds demand. The pathway itself remains intact even in states of depletion, but its throughput is constrained by substrate availability, enzymatic activity, and energy supply. Recovery does not come from forcing the system but from reestablishing alignment across these inputs so that synthesis can scale naturally in response to demand.

The first requirement is restoration of substrate flow, with particular emphasis on cysteine and glycine. Cysteine determines whether synthesis can initiate, and its availability depends on both direct intake and internal conversion pathways that require coordinated nutrient input. Glycine determines whether synthesis can complete and sustain throughput once initiated. Increasing availability of these substrates does not immediately raise glutathione levels, but it removes the constraints that prevent the pathway from operating at full capacity. The system can then begin to rebuild its pool through continuous production rather than intermittent output.

Enzymatic activity must be supported so that available substrates are converted efficiently. Glutamate-cysteine ligase and glutathione synthetase respond to changes in substrate levels and redox state, but their effective output depends on maintaining structural integrity and proper regulation. When these enzymes are operating correctly, increases in substrate availability translate directly into increased production.

When they are impaired, additional substrate does not produce proportional increases in output, and the system remains constrained.

Energy availability determines whether synthesis can proceed at the required rate. Both steps of glutathione construction require ATP, linking production directly to mitochondrial function. Restoring consistent energy output allows the pathway to operate continuously rather than in short, limited bursts. At the same time, NADPH production must be sufficient to maintain recycling of existing glutathione, reducing the pressure on synthesis to replace oxidized molecules. This coordination allows synthesis to expand the pool rather than simply maintain it.

Transport and distribution must support delivery of substrates to the cytosol where synthesis occurs. Amino acids must be available at the site of assembly, and intracellular conditions must allow them to be directed into the synthesis pathway rather than diverted entirely into competing processes. As substrate flow stabilizes, synthesis becomes more consistent and less dependent on transient fluctuations in availability.

Detoxification demand must also be considered during restoration. If reactive load remains high, newly synthesized glutathione is immediately consumed, limiting the ability to expand the pool. Reducing ongoing demand allows synthesis to outpace consumption, creating a net increase in available glutathione. This shift from maintenance to expansion is necessary to rebuild buffering capacity.

Restoration of synthesis capacity is therefore a process of reestablishing system alignment rather than introducing a single input. Substrate availability, enzyme function, energy supply, and demand must operate together so that production can exceed consumption. When these conditions are restored, glutathione synthesis transitions from constrained output to continuous expansion, allowing the system to rebuild its buffering capacity and reestablish stable redox control.

Amino Acid Sufficiency

Amino acid sufficiency defines whether the system has the raw material required to sustain continuous glutathione production under real demand rather than baseline conditions. The pathway depends on glutamate, cysteine, and glycine, but sufficiency is not simply the presence of these amino acids in circulation. It is the ability to maintain their availability at the site of synthesis over time while they are simultaneously being used in multiple competing processes. When supply is consistent and allocation is balanced, synthesis proceeds without interruption. When supply is intermittent or diverted, production becomes constrained even if total intake appears adequate.

Cysteine sets the threshold for initiation because it is maintained at low intracellular concentrations and must be supplied or generated continuously. Sufficiency at this level means that cysteine is available at the moment synthesis is required, not just present in the system in total. If cysteine delivery or conversion from precursor pathways does not match demand, the first step of synthesis slows regardless of glutamate or glycine availability. This creates a condition where the system is structurally intact but unable to begin production at the required rate.

Glycine defines whether synthesis can complete and maintain throughput once initiated. It is distributed across multiple pathways that expand during periods of repair, growth, and increased metabolic activity. Sufficiency requires that glycine supply scales with these competing demands so that enough remains available to finalize glutathione construction. When glycine is drawn into other processes without adequate replenishment, intermediate structures accumulate and output of functional glutathione declines.

Glutamate is less frequently limiting, but its availability still influences the stability of the pathway. It serves as the structural anchor of the molecule and must be present consistently for synthesis to proceed. Fluctuations in glutamate availability can slow the pathway and contribute to variability in production, particularly when other substrates are already constrained.

Amino acid sufficiency is also determined by transport and intracellular distribution. These substrates must be delivered into the cytosol and directed toward the synthesis pathway rather than being fully allocated to protein synthesis, energy metabolism, or signaling functions. When transport is efficient and allocation is balanced, substrates remain available for glutathione production even under increased demand.

The system responds to sufficiency by increasing synthesis output when demand rises. When substrates are available in proportion to need, the pathway scales without interruption and supports expansion of the glutathione pool. When sufficiency is not maintained, synthesis becomes intermittent and cannot keep pace with consumption, forcing the system to rely on recycling alone.

Amino acid sufficiency therefore defines the material foundation of glutathione synthesis. It determines whether the system has continuous access to the components required to build new molecules at a rate that matches or exceeds demand. When this foundation is stable, synthesis supports recovery and expansion of buffering capacity. When it is not, the system operates under constraint, limiting its ability to restore and maintain redox balance.

Enzyme Support

Enzyme support determines whether the glutathione pathway can convert available substrates into functional output at a rate that matches demand. The structure of the pathway is fixed, but its performance depends on how effectively key enzymes operate within current cellular conditions. Glutamate-cysteine ligase controls entry into synthesis, glutathione synthetase completes the molecule, and glutathione reductase restores it after use. If these enzymes are present but operating below capacity, the system remains intact yet underperforms, creating a gap between available resources and actual glutathione output.

Support begins with maintaining the structural integrity of these enzymes so they can sustain catalytic activity. Enzymes require specific intracellular conditions to maintain their active configuration. Oxidative modification, substrate imbalance, or instability in the surrounding environment alters their shape and reduces their ability to bind substrates and carry out reactions. When glutathione levels are already reduced, this creates a reinforcing effect where declining redox control further impairs the enzymes responsible for restoring it.

Cofactor availability plays a direct role in enzyme performance. Glutathione reductase depends on a continuous supply of NADPH to drive reduction of oxidized glutathione. Without sufficient reducing equivalents, the enzyme cannot restore the pool regardless of its presence. Similarly, ATP is required for both steps of glutathione synthesis, linking enzymatic throughput to energy availability. When these inputs are consistent, enzymes operate at rates that match substrate supply. When they are limited, reaction speed declines and the pathway becomes constrained.

Regulatory control also influences enzyme activity. Glutamate-cysteine ligase responds to feedback from existing glutathione levels, increasing activity when the pool is depleted and reducing activity when levels are sufficient. This control mechanism allows the system to adjust production dynamically, but it requires the enzyme to respond accurately to these signals. If responsiveness is reduced, the system loses its ability to scale production in proportion to demand.

Enzyme support is also tied to turnover and maintenance. Enzymes are continually synthesized and degraded, and their replacement must keep pace with functional demand. When protein synthesis is constrained or degradation increases, the total active enzyme pool declines, reducing overall pathway capacity. This creates a condition where substrates are present but cannot be processed efficiently due to insufficient catalytic infrastructure.

The effects of reduced enzyme support extend across both synthesis and recycling. Slower synthesis limits the addition of new glutathione, while slower recycling reduces the availability of existing molecules. Together, these effects reduce total functional capacity and increase reliance on pathways that are already constrained.

Enzyme support therefore defines how effectively the glutathione system can translate substrate availability and energy input into usable buffering capacity. It determines whether the pathway operates at full throughput or remains limited despite adequate inputs. When enzyme activity is maintained, synthesis and recycling align with demand and support system stability. When it is reduced, the pathway becomes a bottleneck, limiting the system's ability to restore and maintain redox balance.

Chapter 25

Reducing Demand

Reducing demand is required when the rate of glutathione consumption exceeds the system's ability to synthesize and recycle it. In this state, increasing production alone does not restore balance because newly generated glutathione is immediately consumed by ongoing reactive load and detoxification pressure. The system remains in a deficit condition where consumption outpaces replacement. Recovery requires lowering the rate at which glutathione is used so that synthesis and recycling can begin to exceed demand and rebuild the pool.

Reactive intermediate production is the primary driver of demand. These intermediates are generated continuously through mitochondrial energy production and are increased when electron flow becomes inefficient. When mitochondrial function is unstable, more electrons escape before completing the transport sequence, forming reactive species that must be neutralized. Reducing this leakage lowers the number of glutathione molecules required for containment. As reactive production decreases, the system shifts from continuous high consumption to a level that can be matched by existing recycling capacity.

Detoxification load contributes a parallel demand on glutathione. Reactive compounds and electrophiles must be conjugated and removed, consuming glutathione in the process. When exposure is high or when partially processed intermediates recirculate, the system diverts a larger portion of its glutathione pool into conjugation and export. Reducing this load decreases the rate at which glutathione is removed from the active pool, allowing more molecules to remain available for redox buffering and reducing the pressure on synthesis.

Incomplete inflammatory cycles increase demand by maintaining a continuous background of reactive signaling. When inflammation does not resolve, reactive intermediates are produced at a sustained level that requires ongoing neutralization. Lowering this persistent activation reduces the continuous drain on the glutathione system and allows recovery processes to operate without constant interruption.

Energy inefficiency further amplifies demand. When ATP production is inconsistent, processes that depend on stable energy input become less efficient, increasing the need for compensatory activity that generates additional reactive intermediates. As energy production stabilizes, the system requires less compensatory throughput, reducing both reactive generation and glutathione consumption.

Demand reduction changes the system from a state of constant depletion to one where recovery becomes possible. As consumption decreases, recycling begins to restore a higher proportion of glutathione to its reduced form, and synthesis can begin to add new molecules to the pool rather than simply replacing what has been lost. This creates a shift where the system moves from maintaining minimal function to rebuilding capacity.

Reducing demand therefore addresses the consumption side of the balance equation. It lowers the rate at which glutathione is used across redox buffering, detoxification, and inflammatory signaling. When demand is brought into alignment with the system's ability to produce and recycle glutathione, the conditions required for restoration are established, allowing the system to transition from deficit to recovery.

Lowering Oxidative Load

Lowering oxidative load reduces the rate at which glutathione is forced into continuous turnover and allows the system to regain control over redox balance. Reactive intermediates are generated as a normal output of metabolism, but when their production rises beyond what can be contained in real time, glutathione is consumed faster than it can be restored. Reducing this load does not eliminate reactive processes.

It brings their rate back into alignment with the system's capacity to neutralize and recover.

The largest contribution to oxidative load comes from mitochondrial electron leakage. When electron flow through the transport system is uneven, a greater portion of electrons escape and form reactive species instead of completing the sequence that produces ATP. Improving the efficiency of this flow reduces leakage at the source, lowering the number of reactive intermediates that must be handled downstream. As leakage declines, glutathione is required less frequently for immediate containment, allowing more of the pool to remain in its reduced, active state.

Substrate handling also influences oxidative load. When substrates are processed cleanly through coordinated pathways, fewer partially oxidized intermediates are generated. When processing becomes disordered, incomplete reactions produce additional reactive species that increase demand on the glutathione system. Stabilizing how substrates enter and move through metabolic pathways reduces the formation of these intermediates and lowers overall reactive pressure.

External inputs contribute to load by introducing compounds that require detoxification. These compounds must be processed through pathways that consume glutathione, increasing turnover even if internal reactive production remains unchanged. Reducing the influx of such compounds decreases the rate at which glutathione is diverted into conjugation and export, preserving more of the pool for redox buffering.

Membrane composition influences how reactive intermediates propagate once they are formed. When membrane structure supports controlled interactions, reactive species are more easily contained and terminated. When membranes are altered, chain reactions spread more readily, increasing the number of events that must be neutralized. Stabilizing membrane composition reduces propagation and limits the expansion of oxidative processes.

Lowering oxidative load changes the system's operating conditions. Instead of responding to a continuous stream of reactive intermediates, the glutathione system handles a level of activity that can be contained and resolved within each cycle. Recycling becomes sufficient to maintain a high proportion of reduced glutathione, and synthesis is no longer required to compensate for constant depletion.

This shift allows the system to move from reactive management to controlled regulation. As load decreases, the balance between oxidation and reduction stabilizes, and glutathione availability increases without requiring excessive production. Lowering oxidative load therefore reduces consumption at its source, creating the conditions necessary for the system to restore and maintain its buffering capacity over time.

Improving Environment

Improving the cellular environment changes how efficiently the glutathione system operates by stabilizing the conditions in which synthesis, recycling, and utilization occur. The pathway itself does not function in isolation. It depends on the physical and chemical state of the intracellular space, including redox balance, pH, ionic gradients, and membrane organization. When these conditions are stable, enzymatic reactions proceed with predictable kinetics and substrates are directed into appropriate pathways. When the environment is unstable, reaction efficiency declines, substrate allocation becomes inconsistent, and glutathione is consumed without restoring balance.

Redox environment is the primary determinant of how the system behaves. A stable ratio between reduced and oxidized molecules allows enzymes involved in synthesis and recycling to operate without interference. When the environment shifts toward a more oxidized state, enzymes become structurally altered and less effective, reducing both production and recovery of glutathione. Restoring a more balanced redox state allows these enzymes to maintain their functional configuration, increasing throughput without requiring additional structural changes to the pathway.

Intracellular pH influences reaction rates and enzyme binding. Glutathione-related enzymes operate within a narrow pH range where substrate affinity and catalytic activity are maintained. Deviations from this range alter enzyme conformation and reduce reaction efficiency.

Stabilizing pH supports consistent enzyme-substrate interaction, allowing synthesis and recycling to proceed at expected rates rather than fluctuating in response to environmental shifts.

Membrane structure determines how substrates and cofactors are transported into and within the cell. Amino acids required for synthesis must cross membranes and reach the cytosol, while NADPH and ATP must be distributed to where they are needed. When membrane composition supports proper transport and compartmentalization, these inputs arrive in a coordinated manner. When membranes are disordered, transport becomes inconsistent, leading to localized shortages that limit pathway throughput even when total availability is sufficient.

Ionic balance and mineral availability influence both enzyme activity and energy production. Enzymatic reactions depend on proper ionic conditions to maintain structure and facilitate binding. Mitochondrial function depends on gradients that drive ATP production, which in turn supports synthesis. Disruption of these gradients reduces energy availability and slows the entire system. Stabilizing ionic conditions supports both the energy supply and the catalytic environment required for glutathione production and recycling.

The extracellular environment also feeds into intracellular stability. Continuous exposure to reactive inputs or fluctuating nutrient availability forces the system to operate under variable conditions, increasing demand and reducing efficiency. Reducing variability in these inputs allows intracellular conditions to stabilize, lowering the need for constant adjustment and preserving glutathione for controlled use rather than emergency response.

Improving environment therefore increases the efficiency of every component of the glutathione system without directly altering the pathway itself. It reduces interference with enzymatic activity, stabilizes substrate delivery, and supports consistent energy production. As these conditions normalize, synthesis and recycling become more effective, consumption becomes more controlled, and the system can maintain redox balance with less strain.

Chapter 26

Supporting Recycling Systems

Supporting recycling systems restores the efficiency with which existing glutathione is returned to its active, reduced form after it has been used. Every cycle of neutralization converts glutathione from its reduced state into an oxidized form that must be converted back before it can participate again. The speed and completeness of this conversion determine how much of the total glutathione pool remains functionally available at any moment. When recycling is efficient, a smaller total pool can sustain high performance because molecules are reused continuously. When recycling slows, the same pool behaves as if it were smaller because a larger fraction remains inactive at any given time.

The central reaction is driven by glutathione reductase, which converts oxidized glutathione back into its reduced form using reducing equivalents supplied by NADPH. This creates a direct dependency between recycling capacity and the availability of NADPH. If NADPH production is stable, oxidized glutathione is rapidly returned to circulation and the system maintains a high proportion of active molecules. If NADPH is limited, oxidized glutathione accumulates, reducing the effective size of the pool and increasing pressure on synthesis to compensate.

NADPH generation is distributed across multiple pathways, with a primary contribution from the pentose phosphate pathway and additional input from mitochondrial and cytosolic reactions that transfer reducing equivalents. The rate at which these pathways operate determines whether recycling can keep pace with demand. When substrate flow through these pathways is consistent and enzymatic activity is maintained, NADPH supply remains sufficient to support continuous recycling. When these pathways are constrained, the system shifts toward a state where oxidation events outpace reduction, and the balance of the pool moves away from its active form.

Energy availability interacts with recycling by determining whether supporting pathways can operate at the required rate. Although the reduction step itself depends on NADPH, the production of NADPH is tied to metabolic activity that requires coordinated energy input. When energy production is unstable, NADPH generation fluctuates, leading to intermittent recycling and periods where oxidized glutathione accumulates. Stabilizing energy output supports consistent NADPH production and maintains continuous recycling.

Recycling capacity also depends on the distribution of glutathione across cellular compartments. Mitochondria, cytosol, and nucleus maintain distinct pools that must each be reduced locally. If recycling is efficient in one compartment but limited in another, localized depletion occurs even when total glutathione appears sufficient. Supporting recycling therefore requires maintaining NADPH availability and enzymatic activity within each compartment so that reduction can occur where oxidation takes place.

The interaction between recycling and synthesis defines overall system efficiency. When recycling is strong, synthesis can focus on expanding the pool rather than replacing oxidized molecules. When recycling is weak, synthesis is diverted into maintaining baseline levels, limiting the system's ability to increase capacity. Strengthening recycling shifts this balance, allowing existing molecules to remain in circulation longer and reducing the total input required to sustain function.

Supporting recycling systems therefore increases the functional lifespan of each glutathione molecule. It ensures that oxidation events do not remove molecules from circulation but instead cycle them back into active use. By maintaining NADPH supply, stabilizing energy production, and supporting enzymatic activity across compartments, the system preserves its existing resources and reduces reliance on continuous synthesis to maintain redox balance.

NADPH and Metabolic Support

NADPH defines whether the glutathione system can maintain a high proportion of its pool in the reduced, functional state under continuous demand. Each time glutathione neutralizes a reactive intermediate, it is converted into an oxidized form that cannot participate again until it is reduced. That reduction step depends directly on NADPH. When NADPH supply is stable, oxidized glutathione is rapidly returned to circulation and the system behaves as a continuously renewing buffer. When NADPH supply falls behind, oxidized glutathione accumulates, shrinking the active pool and forcing synthesis to compensate for what is effectively a recycling failure.

The primary source of NADPH is the pentose phosphate pathway, which diverts glucose-derived intermediates away from energy production and into reducing power generation. This diversion is not optional under oxidative demand. It is a necessary shift that prioritizes redox stability over maximal ATP yield. When substrate flow through this pathway is sufficient and enzyme activity is intact, NADPH production scales with demand and supports continuous recycling. When this flow is limited, either by substrate restriction or impaired pathway activity, NADPH output declines and recycling slows regardless of how much glutathione is present.

Additional NADPH is generated through linked metabolic systems that transfer reducing equivalents between compartments. Mitochondrial reactions contribute to the overall pool by supporting cytosolic reduction indirectly, creating a coordinated network rather than a single-point source. This coordination depends on consistent substrate availability and functional enzyme systems across compartments. Disruption in one area reduces the total reducing capacity available to the system, even if other pathways remain active.

Metabolic support therefore determines whether NADPH production can match the rate at which reducing equivalents are consumed. Substrate availability must be consistent so that NADPH-generating pathways are not forced into intermittent operation. Enzymes within these pathways must maintain structural integrity so that conversion rates remain high enough to meet demand. Energy production must also remain stable, as fluctuations in ATP availability alter how substrates are allocated between energy generation and redox support.

When metabolic support is aligned, NADPH production becomes continuous rather than reactive. Recycling proceeds at the same pace as oxidation, and the majority of the glutathione pool remains in its reduced state. This reduces the burden on synthesis and allows the system to expand its capacity rather than constantly replace what has been lost.

NADPH and metabolic support therefore define the renewal rate of the glutathione system. They determine whether used molecules are rapidly returned to function or accumulate in an inactive state. When NADPH supply is sufficient and stable, recycling maintains the system with minimal loss. When it is not, the system shifts toward depletion, even if total glutathione production remains unchanged.

Chapter 27

Integration with Lipid Systems

Glutathione operates within a lipid-defined environment, and its effectiveness is determined as much by membrane composition as by its own concentration. Reactive intermediates are generated in proximity to membranes and propagate through lipid structures when not contained. The role of glutathione is to intercept and terminate these reactions, but the extent of its workload depends on how easily those reactions spread within the lipid architecture. Membrane composition sets the baseline rate of propagation, while glutathione determines whether that propagation is contained or allowed to expand.

Lipid peroxidation begins when reactive species interact with susceptible fatty acids within membrane phospholipids. This interaction produces lipid radicals that initiate chain reactions, spreading structural damage across the membrane. Glutathione does not act directly on the initial lipid radical. It supports enzymatic systems that convert reactive lipid intermediates into stable forms, terminating the chain reaction before it expands. The efficiency of this process depends on both the availability of glutathione and the susceptibility of the membrane to ongoing propagation.

Membrane composition determines how easily these reactions spread. Polyunsaturated fatty acids are more susceptible to peroxidation due to their chemical structure, allowing chain reactions to propagate more readily once initiated. Saturated and monounsaturated structures resist propagation, limiting the spread of damage even when reactive intermediates are present. When membranes are composed in a way that slows propagation, the number of reactions that must be terminated by glutathione decreases. When membranes are highly susceptible, each initiation event expands into multiple reactions, increasing demand on the glutathione system.

Vitamin E operates within the membrane as a first-line barrier, interrupting lipid peroxidation at the point of propagation. When vitamin E neutralizes a lipid radical, it becomes oxidized and must be restored to continue functioning. Glutathione supports this restoration indirectly by maintaining the redox environment required for vitamin E recycling. This creates a layered defense where membrane-bound antioxidants limit the spread of reactions, and glutathione maintains the conditions that allow those antioxidants to remain active.

Transport between aqueous and lipid environments also defines how these systems interact. Glutathione is primarily located in aqueous compartments, while lipid peroxidation occurs within membranes. The connection between these spaces is mediated by enzymes and intermediate carriers that transfer reactive products out of the membrane for processing. Efficient transfer reduces the time that reactive intermediates remain within the lipid environment, limiting propagation and reducing the total number of reactions that must be managed.

Mitochondrial membranes represent a critical interface where energy production and lipid stability intersect. High electron flow increases the likelihood of reactive intermediate formation near these membranes. If membrane composition supports controlled propagation and glutathione recycling is efficient, these reactions are contained without disrupting energy production. If either condition is compromised, lipid peroxidation spreads, altering membrane properties and further destabilizing electron transport.

Integration with lipid systems therefore defines the scale of the problem that glutathione must solve. Membrane composition sets the rate and spread of reactive processes, while glutathione determines whether those processes are contained and resolved. When both systems are aligned, reactive events remain localized and manageable. When they are not, small initiation events expand into widespread damage, increasing demand on glutathione and accelerating depletion of the system.

Membrane Protection

Membrane protection is where glutathione's role becomes structural rather than purely chemical, because the integrity of the membrane determines how signals move, how gradients are maintained, and how the cell preserves separation between internal and external environments. Every membrane is built from lipid assemblies that must remain stable under continuous exposure to reactive intermediates generated during normal metabolism. When these lipids are altered, the membrane changes behavior. Permeability shifts, embedded proteins lose alignment, and signaling becomes less controlled. Glutathione functions to limit these alterations by constraining the reactions that would otherwise propagate across the lipid structure.

The primary threat to membranes is the spread of lipid peroxidation. A single reactive interaction with a susceptible fatty acid can initiate a chain reaction that moves laterally through the membrane, altering multiple lipid molecules in sequence. This process does not remain localized unless it is actively terminated. Glutathione supports the enzymatic systems that intercept these intermediates and convert them into stable forms before they continue propagating. The speed of this interception determines whether the event remains isolated or expands into broader structural disruption.

Membrane composition directly affects how much work glutathione must perform. Lipids that are more resistant to peroxidation limit the ability of chain reactions to spread, reducing the number of reactive intermediates that need to be neutralized. In this state, glutathione operates as a control mechanism that resolves isolated events. When membranes contain a higher proportion of easily oxidized lipids, each initiation event generates multiple downstream reactions, increasing the total number of intermediates that must be processed. This shifts glutathione from a control role into a constant containment role, increasing consumption and accelerating depletion.

Membrane proteins depend on lipid stability to maintain their position and function. Receptors, transporters, and enzymes embedded in the membrane require a consistent lipid environment to operate correctly. When lipid structure is altered, these proteins change conformation or lose efficiency, disrupting transport and signaling processes. Glutathione contributes to preserving this environment by limiting the oxidative modifications that would otherwise alter lipid organization and protein behavior.

Energy production is directly tied to membrane integrity within mitochondria. The gradients that drive ATP synthesis depend on tightly controlled membrane properties. Lipid peroxidation disrupts these properties, allowing leakage that reduces efficiency and increases reactive intermediate generation. This creates a feedback loop where membrane damage increases oxidative load, which in turn accelerates further damage. By supporting the containment of lipid peroxidation, glutathione helps preserve the conditions required for stable energy production.

Membrane protection therefore represents a convergence point between structure and function. Glutathione does not rebuild membranes directly, but it determines whether the existing structure remains intact long enough for normal maintenance processes to keep pace. When protection is sufficient, membranes retain their organization, signaling remains precise, and energy systems operate efficiently. When it is not, structural instability spreads, increasing system-wide demand and reducing the cell's ability to maintain controlled function.

Interaction with Omega-3 and Vitamin E

The interaction between glutathione, omega-3 lipids, and vitamin E forms a layered system that controls how membranes behave under oxidative pressure. Each component operates in a different physical space but they are functionally linked. Omega-3 fatty acids integrate into membrane phospholipids and alter the physical structure of the membrane, vitamin E resides within the lipid layer and intercepts propagating reactions, and glutathione operates in the aqueous environment supporting the restoration and termination processes that allow the system to reset after each event. The outcome depends on how these layers coordinate rather than on the presence of any single component.

Omega-3 fatty acids change membrane properties by increasing fluidity and altering how proteins and signaling complexes are organized within the lipid bilayer. This affects receptor behavior, transport dynamics, and how signals are transmitted across the membrane. At the same time, their chemical structure makes them more susceptible to interaction with reactive intermediates. This does not create a problem on its own, but it increases the requirement for a functioning containment system. When omega-3 content rises, the system must be able to manage a higher probability of lipid interaction without allowing chain reactions to propagate.

Vitamin E functions at the point where these reactions would otherwise spread. It intercepts lipid radicals within the membrane and terminates the chain reaction by donating an electron, preventing further propagation across adjacent lipids. This action converts vitamin E into an oxidized form that cannot continue functioning until it is restored. The rate at which vitamin E is recycled determines whether it remains available to perform this role continuously or becomes depleted after repeated use.

Glutathione supports this restoration indirectly by maintaining the redox environment required for vitamin E to be returned to its active state. It does not interact with the lipid radical directly but enables the systems that transfer reducing equivalents back to oxidized vitamin E. When glutathione levels are sufficient and recycling is active, vitamin E remains in circulation within the membrane, repeatedly intercepting propagation events. When glutathione is depleted, vitamin E accumulates in its oxidized form, reducing the effectiveness of this first-line defense and allowing lipid peroxidation to spread more easily.

This interaction creates a dependency between membrane composition and redox capacity. Increasing omega-3 content without maintaining vitamin E and glutathione support raises the likelihood that initiation events will propagate beyond control. Maintaining all three components in alignment allows membranes to incorporate omega-3 fatty acids while still containing reactive processes efficiently. In this state, omega-3 integration contributes to signaling and structural function without increasing net oxidative burden.

The system operates as a sequence. Reactive intermediates interact with membrane lipids, vitamin E intercepts and stops the spread, and glutathione-dependent systems restore vitamin E so the process can repeat. If any step slows or fails, the sequence breaks, and propagation expands. The result is not a localized event but a widening area of membrane alteration that increases overall demand on the system.

The interaction between omega-3, vitamin E, and glutathione therefore defines whether membrane remodeling leads to improved function or increased instability. When these components are balanced, membranes remain responsive and controlled under oxidative conditions. When they are not, structural changes increase vulnerability, and the burden shifts onto glutathione to contain reactions that could have been limited at the membrane level.

Chapter 28

Supplementation

Supplementation enters the system as an external attempt to modify glutathione availability, but its effectiveness depends entirely on how it interfaces with the existing architecture of synthesis, recycling, and demand. The system does not treat supplementation as a direct override. It processes these inputs through the same pathways that govern endogenous production and utilization. Whether supplementation produces a measurable effect depends on whether it removes an existing constraint or simply adds material that cannot be efficiently integrated.

Direct Glutathione vs Precursor-Based Strategies

Direct glutathione delivery and precursor-based strategies enter the system at different points in the pathway, and their outcomes are determined by how well they align with the body's existing architecture for synthesis, transport, and recycling. Delivering glutathione introduces the completed molecule, while precursor strategies supply the components required to build it internally. The distinction is not just chemical. It defines whether the system is being supplemented at the endpoint or supported at the level where control is exerted.

Direct glutathione faces immediate constraints once it enters circulation. Outside the cell, glutathione is subject to breakdown, and its intact transfer into intracellular compartments is limited. Even when delivery systems improve stability and transport, the molecule must still be distributed into specific cellular compartments where it can participate in redox control. If distribution is uneven or if intracellular retention is low, the added glutathione contributes to transient increases in availability but does not significantly expand the functional pool. It becomes part of ongoing turnover, entering and exiting the system without shifting baseline capacity.

Precursor-based strategies operate within the system's native construction pathway. By supplying cysteine and glycine, they allow glutathione to be synthesized directly in the cytosol where it is needed. This approach uses existing enzymatic control, meaning production increases in proportion to demand when substrates are available. The system determines how much glutathione to produce based on current conditions, and precursor availability removes the constraints that would otherwise limit that response. This results in a more stable increase in intracellular levels rather than a temporary external input.

The effectiveness of precursor strategies depends on whether both initiation and completion steps are supported. Cysteine controls entry into the pathway, while glycine determines whether synthesis can proceed to completion. Supplying one without the other creates an imbalance where intermediates accumulate and final output remains limited. When both substrates are available in sufficient amounts, synthesis becomes continuous and capable of expanding the pool rather than simply maintaining it.

Recycling capacity influences both strategies but becomes more critical for direct glutathione. If recycling is efficient, delivered glutathione can be reused after oxidation, extending its functional lifespan. If recycling is limited, delivered glutathione is quickly converted into its oxidized form and not restored, reducing the duration of its effect. Precursor strategies partially offset this by allowing the system to replace oxidized molecules through synthesis, but they still depend on recycling to maintain efficiency.

System demand ultimately determines which approach produces a meaningful change. When demand is high, direct glutathione is rapidly consumed, and precursor-based synthesis must be able to scale to keep pace. When demand is controlled and recycling is functional, precursor strategies allow the system to build and maintain a larger pool over time. Direct delivery may still provide short-term increases, but without integration into the system's internal processes, those increases do not persist.

Direct glutathione and precursor-based strategies therefore represent two different ways of interacting with the same system. One attempts to supply the end product, while the other supports the system's ability to produce it. Long-term changes in capacity depend on whether the system can continuously generate and recycle glutathione internally. When that capacity is restored, precursor strategies align with system function and produce sustained effects, while direct delivery remains a secondary input that is limited by distribution and turnover.

Absorption, Stability, and Delivery Systems (Liposomal, S-Acetyl)

Absorption and stability determine how much of a supplemented compound reaches the point where it can be used, while delivery systems determine how it moves through the body and into cells. Glutathione is particularly sensitive to these constraints because it is reactive and structurally vulnerable outside the intracellular environment where it normally functions. When administered directly, a significant portion is altered or broken down before it can contribute to intracellular pools, which limits the effectiveness of simple oral delivery.

Stability is the first limiting factor. In aqueous and digestive environments, glutathione can be degraded or modified before absorption occurs. This reduces the fraction that remains intact long enough to cross into circulation. Even after absorption, it must persist long enough to reach target tissues without being rapidly consumed or converted. Forms that increase structural stability extend the time window in which glutathione remains intact, improving the likelihood that it reaches cells in a usable form.

Delivery systems attempt to address transport across membranes, which is a second major constraint. Glutathione does not freely diffuse into cells at high rates, so delivery approaches aim to alter how it interacts with cellular membranes. Liposomal systems encapsulate glutathione within lipid structures that resemble portions of the cell membrane. This allows the compound to move through lipid environments more effectively and increases the probability of intracellular delivery. Once inside, glutathione must still integrate into the existing pool and enter normal recycling and utilization pathways.

S-acetyl glutathione modifies the molecule to increase its resistance to breakdown during absorption. This structural change protects reactive sites, allowing more of the administered compound to remain intact during transit. After absorption, the modification must be removed to release active glutathione within the cell. The efficiency of this conversion determines how much of the delivered compound becomes functionally available.

These delivery systems increase the fraction of administered glutathione that reaches intracellular compartments, but they do not change how the system processes it once it arrives. The molecule still enters the same redox cycle, is subject to the same recycling constraints, and is consumed at the same rate under oxidative demand. If recycling capacity is limited or demand remains high, improved delivery increases input without changing overall system balance.

Absorption efficiency also interacts with dosing patterns. Higher bioavailability allows smaller amounts to achieve measurable intracellular presence, while lower bioavailability requires larger inputs to reach similar levels. However, increasing dose does not overcome limitations in transport, recycling, or demand. Excess amounts may circulate transiently or be cleared without contributing to sustained increases in functional glutathione.

Delivery systems therefore improve access to the intracellular environment but do not replace the need for system alignment. They increase the efficiency of getting glutathione into the system, but the outcome still depends on how well synthesis, recycling, and demand are coordinated. When these systems are functioning, improved delivery contributes to expansion of the glutathione pool. When they are not, it produces temporary increases in availability without altering long-term capacity.

Cysteine and Glycine Repletion (NAC, Glycine, Protein Sources)

Cysteine and glycine repletion restores the substrate layer of the glutathione system, allowing synthesis to proceed without interruption and at a rate that can match demand. The pathway is structurally simple, but its throughput is controlled by whether these amino acids are available at the point of synthesis in the cytosol. When either is limited, production slows or stalls regardless of enzyme presence or energy availability. Repletion is not defined by total intake alone. It requires consistent delivery, intracellular availability, and allocation toward the synthesis pathway rather than competing uses.

Cysteine defines entry into the pathway. It is maintained at low intracellular levels and is rapidly consumed when demand increases, making it the most common limiting substrate. Direct cysteine is unstable in circulation, so it is often supplied through precursors such as N-acetylcysteine, which are converted into cysteine within the cell. This conversion depends on enzymatic activity and the availability of cofactors that support sulfur metabolism. When conversion is efficient, cysteine supply becomes continuous and initiation of synthesis proceeds without delay. When conversion is constrained, increasing precursor intake does not translate into higher intracellular cysteine at the point of use.

Glycine determines whether synthesis can complete and sustain throughput after initiation. It is used across multiple systems, including protein synthesis, detoxification, and structural maintenance, and demand for glycine expands during repair and metabolic stress. Repletion requires that supply is sufficient to meet these competing demands while still allowing glutathione synthesis to proceed. When glycine availability is marginal, intermediate compounds accumulate and final glutathione output remains limited even if cysteine is present.

Protein sources provide a broader substrate base by supplying all required amino acids along with additional components that support overall metabolic function. Intact protein delivers cysteine and glycine within a matrix that also contributes to enzyme turnover and repair processes. The rate at which these amino acids become available depends on digestion and absorption efficiency, which influences how consistently substrates are delivered into circulation and ultimately into cells.

Transport into the cell and allocation within it determine whether repleted substrates are used for glutathione synthesis. Amino acids must cross membranes and reach the cytosol, where they compete with other pathways for utilization. When transport systems are functioning and intracellular conditions are stable, a portion of these substrates is directed into glutathione production. When transport is inconsistent or demand from other pathways is high, available amino acids are diverted away from synthesis, limiting output despite adequate intake.

Repletion becomes effective when both substrates are present in sufficient amounts and delivered consistently enough to support continuous synthesis. The pathway then operates without interruption, allowing the glutathione pool to expand rather than simply maintain baseline levels. When either substrate remains limiting, production fluctuates and cannot keep pace with consumption.

Cysteine and glycine repletion therefore rebuilds the material foundation of the glutathione system. It determines whether the pathway has access to the components required to produce new molecules at a rate that matches or exceeds demand. When this foundation is restored and aligned with enzyme activity and recycling capacity, synthesis becomes continuous and supports recovery of redox balance.

Sulfur Metabolism and Transsulfuration Support

Sulfur metabolism determines whether cysteine can be generated, maintained, and delivered into the glutathione synthesis pathway under continuous demand. Cysteine does not exist in large reserve pools, and its availability depends on a dynamic balance between intake, conversion, and utilization. The transsulfuration pathway provides a controlled route for converting upstream sulfur-containing amino acids into cysteine, linking overall amino acid metabolism to glutathione production. When this pathway is functioning at sufficient throughput, cysteine supply becomes continuous and responsive to demand. When it is constrained, glutathione synthesis is limited at its point of entry regardless of total sulfur intake.

The pathway begins with methionine, which is activated and processed through a sequence that generates homocysteine. Homocysteine represents a branch point. It can be recycled back into methionine or directed into transsulfuration to produce cysteine. The decision at this branch is influenced by substrate levels, enzyme activity, and the availability of cofactors that support each direction. When transsulfuration is favored and supported, homocysteine is converted through intermediate steps into cysteine, providing a sustained internal source of substrate for glutathione synthesis.

Enzymatic control within this pathway determines its effective output. The conversion steps require specific enzymes that depend on stable intracellular conditions and adequate cofactor support. When enzyme activity is high, the pathway can increase cysteine production in response to demand. When activity is reduced, the flow of sulfur into cysteine slows, creating a bottleneck that limits glutathione synthesis even if upstream substrates are present.

Cofactors define whether these reactions proceed at sufficient rates. The enzymes that drive transsulfuration require consistent availability of vitamins that maintain their structure and catalytic function. When these cofactors are limited, the pathway does not stop completely, but its throughput decreases, reducing cysteine output and constraining downstream synthesis. This creates a condition where sulfur intake appears adequate, but conversion into usable cysteine at the point of synthesis is insufficient.

Sulfur utilization extends beyond glutathione production. Cysteine is also required for protein structure, enzyme function, and other metabolic processes that expand during periods of stress and repair. Increased demand in these areas competes with glutathione synthesis for available cysteine. Transsulfuration must therefore produce enough cysteine to meet multiple simultaneous demands. When production cannot scale, glutathione synthesis is deprioritized, and the system shifts toward maintaining essential structural functions.

Transport and intracellular handling determine whether newly generated cysteine reaches the cytosol where synthesis occurs. Efficient movement and allocation ensure that cysteine produced through transsulfuration contributes directly to glutathione production rather than being fully consumed by competing pathways. When transport is disrupted or allocation is imbalanced, cysteine availability at the synthesis site remains limited despite adequate upstream production.

Transsulfuration support therefore ensures that cysteine supply is not dependent solely on direct intake but can be generated internally in response to demand. It connects sulfur metabolism to redox capacity by controlling how much substrate enters the glutathione pathway. When this system is aligned, cysteine availability becomes continuous and scalable, allowing synthesis to operate without interruption. When it is not, the pathway becomes a limiting factor, restricting the system's ability to restore and maintain glutathione levels.

NADPH and Metabolic Cofactor Support (Riboflavin, Selenium)

NADPH and cofactor availability determine whether the glutathione system can sustain continuous recycling and enzymatic activity under real demand. Glutathione is not consumed in a single pass and discarded. It is cycled repeatedly between reduced and oxidized states, and that cycle depends on a steady supply of reducing equivalents and functional enzymes. NADPH provides the reducing force that restores oxidized glutathione, while specific cofactors maintain the structure and catalytic capacity of the enzymes that carry out both reduction and detoxification. When either side is limited, the system slows even if total glutathione production appears sufficient.

NADPH is generated through metabolic pathways that divert substrates away from energy production and into reducing capacity. This shift is required when oxidative demand rises because maintaining redox balance becomes a priority over maximizing ATP output. The rate of NADPH generation must match the rate at which glutathione is oxidized. When production is consistent, oxidized glutathione is rapidly converted back into its reduced form and re-enters circulation. When NADPH supply falls behind, oxidized glutathione accumulates, reducing the proportion of the pool that is functionally active and increasing reliance on synthesis to compensate.

Riboflavin supports this system by maintaining the functional state of enzymes that transfer reducing equivalents. It is required for the formation of flavin-based cofactors that allow enzymes such as glutathione reductase to accept and pass electrons efficiently. When riboflavin availability is sufficient, these enzymes maintain high catalytic turnover, and NADPH can be used effectively to restore glutathione. When it is limited, enzyme activity declines, and even adequate NADPH cannot be fully utilized, slowing the recycling process.

Selenium supports the enzymes that use glutathione to neutralize reactive intermediates. Glutathione peroxidase relies on selenium to convert reactive species into stable forms, transferring the oxidative burden onto glutathione in a controlled manner. This process determines how efficiently reactive intermediates are neutralized and how much glutathione is required for each event. When selenium-dependent enzyme activity is sufficient, reactions are completed efficiently, limiting unnecessary consumption of glutathione. When it is reduced, reactive intermediates persist longer, increasing the number of interactions that must be managed and accelerating glutathione turnover.

The interaction between NADPH supply and cofactor-supported enzymes defines overall system efficiency. NADPH provides the capacity to restore glutathione, riboflavin ensures that reduction reactions proceed at high speed, and selenium ensures that oxidative reactions are handled efficiently so that glutathione is used in a controlled manner. If any of these components are limited, the system compensates by increasing turnover, which raises demand and reduces stability.

Metabolic alignment determines whether these inputs operate continuously. Substrate availability must support NADPH generation without interruption, and cofactors must be present at levels that sustain enzyme activity over time. When aligned, recycling becomes efficient, enzyme systems operate at full capacity, and glutathione remains in its reduced state for a greater proportion of time. When misaligned, recycling slows, consumption increases, and the system shifts toward depletion despite adequate input.

NADPH and metabolic cofactor support therefore define how effectively the glutathione system can renew itself and process oxidative load. They determine whether each molecule is used once or cycled repeatedly, and whether reactions are completed efficiently or left partially resolved. When these elements are in place, the system maintains high functional capacity with lower total input. When they are not, the system becomes dependent on continuous replacement, limiting its ability to restore and sustain redox balance.

Stack Design and Pathway Coordination

Stack design determines whether multiple inputs converge into a functional increase in glutathione capacity or remain as disconnected interventions that fail to shift system behavior. The glutathione system is not a single pathway that can be forced with one input. It is a coordinated network of substrate supply, enzymatic conversion, energy support, recycling, and demand management. When a stack is constructed without regard to this structure, inputs accumulate without producing a proportional increase in output. When it is aligned with the pathway, each component reinforces the others and total system capacity increases.

Coordination begins at the level of substrate flow. Cysteine and glycine must be present together and delivered consistently so that synthesis can initiate and complete without interruption. Supplying one without the other creates a partial pathway that cannot produce full output. Protein intake, precursor compounds, and sulfur metabolism support must be aligned so that cysteine is continuously available while glycine is not diverted entirely into competing processes. When this layer is coordinated, synthesis becomes stable rather than intermittent.

Enzymatic throughput must match substrate availability. Providing substrates without supporting enzyme function results in accumulation without conversion. Cofactors that maintain enzyme structure and catalytic efficiency allow the pathway to translate substrate input into actual glutathione production. This ensures that increases in availability lead to increases in output rather than unused intermediates.

Recycling must be integrated into the stack so that newly produced or delivered glutathione remains in circulation. NADPH generation and cofactor support determine whether oxidized glutathione is returned to its reduced form or accumulates in an inactive state. When recycling is aligned with synthesis, the system uses each molecule multiple times, reducing the total input required to maintain capacity. When it is not, synthesis is forced into continuous replacement rather than expansion.

Demand management is the controlling variable that determines whether the stack produces a net gain. If oxidative load and detoxification pressure remain high, all inputs are directed toward maintaining baseline function. Lowering demand allows the combined effects of substrate supply, enzyme activity, and recycling to exceed consumption, creating a surplus that expands the glutathione pool. Without this alignment, even well-constructed stacks operate in a deficit condition.

Timing and dosing influence how these components interact. Inputs must be delivered in a pattern that matches how the system processes them. Large, infrequent doses can exceed transport and enzymatic capacity, while consistent input allows steady integration into ongoing pathways. Coordination over time ensures that each layer of the system remains supported rather than oscillating between surplus and deficiency.

Stack design therefore operates as a system-level problem rather than a collection of individual supplements. It requires alignment across substrate availability, enzyme function, recycling capacity, and demand. When these elements are coordinated, the system shifts from constrained throughput to continuous operation, allowing glutathione levels to rise and stabilize. When they are not, inputs remain isolated, and the system continues to operate under the same limitations regardless of how much is added.

Dosing Strategies Based on System State

Dosing strategy determines whether supplementation integrates into the glutathione system or disrupts it by exceeding the capacity of transport, conversion, and recycling pathways. The system does not respond linearly to increasing input. It processes substrates and compounds at rates defined by enzyme activity, energy availability, and current demand. Effective dosing therefore depends on matching input to system state rather than applying fixed amounts independent of underlying conditions.

In a depleted state, the system is operating with limited substrate availability, reduced recycling capacity, and elevated demand. Large inputs introduced into this environment are rapidly consumed or diverted without producing a sustained increase in functional glutathione. Initial dosing in this state must prioritize restoring continuous substrate availability and supporting recycling rather than attempting to elevate levels immediately. Smaller, consistent inputs allow the system to begin rebuilding synthesis capacity and restoring redox balance without overwhelming constrained pathways.

As substrate sufficiency improves and recycling begins to stabilize, dosing can shift toward supporting expansion of the glutathione pool. At this stage, the system is capable of converting additional input into increased output because enzymatic throughput and NADPH availability are no longer primary bottlenecks. Inputs can be increased gradually, allowing synthesis to operate at higher rates while recycling maintains a larger proportion of the pool in its reduced form.

In a stable state, where synthesis, recycling, and demand are aligned, dosing becomes maintenance-focused. The objective is to match ongoing consumption rather than drive further expansion. Inputs are adjusted to maintain consistent substrate availability and support enzyme function without introducing excess that cannot be efficiently utilized. This maintains system equilibrium and prevents unnecessary fluctuations in glutathione levels.

System state also determines how different forms of supplementation are used. In depleted conditions, precursor strategies are prioritized because they rebuild internal production capacity. As the system stabilizes, direct glutathione or enhanced delivery systems can be used to support existing pools without relying entirely on synthesis. The balance between these approaches shifts as the system moves from constraint to stability.

Frequency of dosing influences integration into metabolic pathways. Continuous or repeated smaller doses maintain steady substrate and cofactor availability, supporting consistent pathway activity. Large, infrequent doses create transient spikes that exceed processing capacity, leading to partial utilization and increased clearance without sustained benefit. Matching dosing frequency to the system's ability to process inputs ensures that supplementation contributes to ongoing function rather than temporary elevation.

Demand must be considered alongside dosing. If oxidative load and detoxification pressure remain high, increased input is directed toward maintaining baseline function rather than expanding capacity. Adjusting dosing without addressing demand leads to higher turnover without net gain. Aligning dosing with reduced demand allows input to exceed consumption and produce measurable increases in glutathione levels.

Dosing strategies therefore function as a control mechanism that aligns external input with internal capacity. They determine whether supplementation is converted into sustained increases in functional glutathione or dissipates within existing turnover. When dosing is matched to system state, inputs are integrated efficiently, supporting recovery, expansion, and maintenance as the system progresses through different stages of function.

Failure Points: When Supplementation Cannot Overcome Upstream Constraints

Supplementation fails when it is introduced into a system where the limiting factor sits upstream of the point of intervention. The glutathione system is organized as a sequence of dependencies, and increasing input at one level does not produce output if earlier steps remain constrained. In these conditions, added compounds move through the system without changing its baseline behavior. They are absorbed, processed, and often consumed, but they do not increase functional capacity because the bottleneck has not been removed.

Substrate limitation is the most direct failure point. Supplying glutathione or its precursors does not increase synthesis if cysteine or glycine availability at the cellular level remains inconsistent. This can occur when intake appears sufficient but transport, conversion, or allocation prevents these amino acids from reaching the cytosol in usable amounts. The pathway receives intermittent input, and production remains constrained despite higher total supply. The result is variability in glutathione levels without a sustained increase.

Enzymatic constraints create a second layer of limitation. If glutamate-cysteine ligase, glutathione synthetase, or glutathione reductase are operating below capacity, additional substrate or direct glutathione does not translate into higher functional output. Reaction rates remain fixed by enzyme activity, and excess input accumulates transiently or is diverted into other pathways. In this state, supplementation increases throughput without increasing net capacity, and the system continues to operate below its potential.

Recycling failure limits how long glutathione remains usable once it has been oxidized. When NADPH supply is insufficient or when cofactors required for enzyme activity are limited, oxidized glutathione accumulates and is not efficiently restored. Supplementation adds to the total pool, but a larger fraction of that pool remains inactive. The system behaves as if it is depleted even when total glutathione content is higher, because the proportion available for redox buffering is reduced.

Excess demand overrides supplementation by increasing consumption faster than input can be integrated. High oxidative load, persistent detoxification pressure, and unresolved inflammatory signaling continuously draw on the glutathione pool. In this state, added glutathione or increased synthesis is immediately consumed, preventing expansion of capacity. The system remains in a steady state of high turnover where input and consumption rise together without altering overall balance.

Energy limitation introduces a broader constraint that affects both synthesis and recycling. ATP is required for glutathione construction, and NADPH generation depends on stable metabolic function. When energy production is inconsistent, both processes slow, reducing the system's ability to utilize supplemental input. Compounds enter the system, but conversion and renewal do not keep pace, limiting their effect.

Transport and distribution also determine whether supplementation reaches the compartments where it is needed. If delivery into cells or specific organelles is inefficient, compounds remain in circulation or are cleared without contributing to intracellular pools. Even with improved delivery systems, uneven distribution can create localized deficiencies that persist despite adequate systemic levels.

Failure therefore reflects a mismatch between where supplementation is applied and where the system is constrained. Increasing input at the endpoint does not compensate for limitations in substrate supply, enzyme activity, recycling capacity, energy production, or demand. Effective intervention requires identifying the primary constraint and aligning input to remove it. When that alignment is achieved, supplementation integrates into the system and produces measurable change. When it is not, supplementation remains an isolated input that does not alter underlying function.

PART IX

SYSTEM REINTEGRATION

Returning the body to stable function

Chapter 29

Rebuilding Completion Capacity

Completion capacity defines whether the system can carry a process from initiation through resolution without leaving residual intermediates behind. In the context of glutathione, this means neutralizing reactive species, restoring redox balance, processing byproducts, and returning all participating molecules to a functional state before the next cycle begins. When completion capacity is intact, each cycle closes cleanly and the system resets to baseline. When it is reduced, partial reactions accumulate, and the system begins each new cycle with unresolved material from the previous one.

Rebuilding this capacity requires restoring alignment across synthesis, recycling, and demand so that each stage of the cycle can proceed without interruption. The system must have sufficient glutathione available at the moment of need, must be able to regenerate it after use, and must not be overwhelmed by a rate of reactive input that exceeds its ability to process. If any of these conditions are not met, reactions remain incomplete and intermediates persist.

The first step is restoring continuous availability of reduced glutathione. This depends on stable substrate supply and functional synthesis so that the pool can be maintained at a level that supports real-time buffering. Intermittent production leads to gaps in availability where reactive intermediates are not neutralized immediately, increasing the likelihood of secondary reactions that expand system demand. Continuous synthesis removes these gaps and allows the system to respond without delay.

Recycling must operate at a rate that matches oxidation. Each neutralization event converts glutathione into its oxidized form, and failure to restore it reduces the effective size of the pool. When NADPH supply and enzyme activity are sufficient, oxidized glutathione is rapidly converted back and re-enters circulation. This allows the same molecules to participate in multiple cycles, increasing overall efficiency and supporting completion of each reaction sequence.

Demand must be reduced to a level that can be fully processed within each cycle. When reactive load remains high, even a functional synthesis and recycling system is forced into continuous throughput without achieving closure. Lowering demand allows the system to complete each sequence before the next begins, preventing accumulation of intermediates and restoring a stable baseline.

Compartmental coordination is required so that completion occurs where reactions take place. Each cellular compartment maintains its own glutathione pool and must be able to process local reactive events. If one compartment is limited, incomplete reactions persist in that location even if overall glutathione levels appear sufficient. Rebuilding completion capacity requires ensuring that synthesis, recycling, and availability are aligned across compartments rather than concentrated in a single pool.

As completion capacity is restored, the system transitions from accumulation to resolution. Reactive intermediates are neutralized and cleared within the same cycle in which they are generated. Byproducts are processed and removed, and glutathione is returned to its reduced form before being used again. This reduces background load and prevents the gradual buildup of damage that characterizes a system operating under constraint.

Rebuilding completion capacity therefore represents a shift from partial processing to full resolution. It is not defined by increasing glutathione levels alone but by restoring the system's ability to carry reactions through to completion across synthesis, utilization, and recovery. When this capacity is in place, the system maintains stability over time, preventing accumulation and supporting consistent function under varying conditions.

Detox Completion

Detox completion defines whether compounds entering the system are fully processed, conjugated, and removed, or whether they remain partially transformed and recirculate through the body. The detoxification sequence operates as a staged process where initial modification increases reactivity, conjugation neutralizes that reactivity, and transport systems remove the final product. Glutathione sits at the center of the conjugation phase, where it binds reactive intermediates and converts them into forms that can be safely exported. Completion depends on whether this sequence proceeds without interruption from entry to clearance.

The first stage increases the number of reactive intermediates that must be managed. These compounds are generated as part of normal metabolism and from external inputs, and they are often more reactive after initial processing than before. If conjugation capacity is insufficient at this point, these intermediates persist and interact with cellular structures, increasing system-wide demand. Detox completion therefore requires that glutathione availability matches the rate at which these intermediates are produced, allowing immediate binding and neutralization before secondary interactions occur.

Conjugation converts reactive compounds into stable complexes that are no longer able to participate in damaging reactions. This process consumes glutathione, transferring the reactive burden onto the molecule itself. The efficiency of this step determines how quickly intermediates are neutralized and how much glutathione is required for each event. When conjugation is efficient, intermediates are rapidly converted and prepared for removal. When it is limited, intermediates accumulate, and glutathione is consumed without achieving full neutralization.

Transport and clearance define whether detoxification is completed or stalled at the conjugation stage. Once compounds are bound to glutathione, they must be moved out of the cell and ultimately excreted. If transport systems are functioning, these complexes are removed in a coordinated flow that prevents accumulation. If transport is impaired, conjugated compounds remain within the system, and in some cases can be broken down and re-released as reactive intermediates. This creates a cycle where the same compounds require repeated processing, increasing demand without achieving resolution.

Recycling intersects with detox completion by determining whether glutathione used in conjugation is replaced or restored. When recycling capacity is high and synthesis is active, the system can sustain continuous detoxification without depleting its pool. When recycling is limited, glutathione is removed from circulation through conjugation faster than it can be restored, reducing availability for subsequent cycles and impairing completion.

Energy and substrate availability influence every stage of this sequence. Conjugation requires sufficient glutathione, transport requires functional membrane systems and energy-dependent processes, and clearance depends on coordinated flow through elimination pathways. Disruption at any point slows the entire sequence, allowing intermediates to persist and increasing the likelihood of recirculation.

Detox completion therefore reflects whether the system can carry compounds through the full sequence from modification to removal without leaving reactive material behind. It is defined by alignment across conjugation capacity, transport efficiency, recycling, and demand. When these elements are coordinated, compounds are processed once and removed. When they are not, partial processing becomes the dominant pattern, increasing system load and preventing restoration of stable function.

Immune Resolution

Immune resolution defines whether an activated immune response can return to baseline after the initiating signal has been processed. Activation is not the limiting step. The system is designed to detect disruption and respond rapidly through signaling cascades that increase reactive output, recruit immune cells, and alter local tissue conditions. Resolution requires that these processes shut down once the task is complete, and that shutdown depends on redox conditions that allow signaling pathways to terminate cleanly. Glutathione sits at the center of this transition by controlling the intracellular environment in which these signals either persist or decay.

During activation, reactive intermediates are used as signaling molecules that amplify the immune response. Their presence increases transcription of inflammatory mediators, maintains immune cell recruitment, and sustains the metabolic state required for defense. These signals are not self-limiting. They require active reduction and removal to terminate. When glutathione is available and recycling is efficient, these reactive signals are neutralized after they have served their function, allowing transcriptional activity to decline and immune cells to disengage.

Resolution depends on the ability to shift from a high-reactivity state back to controlled baseline conditions. This shift requires that oxidized signaling components are returned to their reduced forms and that reactive intermediates no longer accumulate. When glutathione levels are sufficient, this transition occurs within the same cycle as activation. The system increases activity, processes the signal, and then returns to baseline without residual activation.

When glutathione is limited, reactive signaling persists beyond its useful window. Transcription factors remain active, inflammatory mediators continue to be produced, and immune cells remain engaged in the absence of a clear target. This creates a condition where the response is no longer proportional to the initiating signal. Instead of a contained event, the system enters a sustained activation state that increases overall demand and disrupts normal tissue function.

Energy and substrate availability influence how quickly resolution can occur. Immune cells require energy to disengage and to transition back to a resting state. Redox conditions must support this transition by allowing signaling pathways to deactivate. If energy production is unstable or if redox balance is not restored, the system remains locked in an activated configuration.

Compartmental control is also required. Resolution must occur locally within tissues where activation took place. If glutathione availability is uneven across compartments, some areas return to baseline while others remain activated. This creates localized persistence of inflammation that can propagate into broader system instability.

Immune resolution therefore depends on the system's ability to terminate its own signaling processes. Glutathione enables this by restoring the redox conditions required for signaling pathways to shut down and for immune activity to return to baseline. When this capacity is intact, immune responses are discrete and self-limited. When it is not, activation extends beyond its intended duration, increasing demand and preventing full recovery of system stability.Chapter 30 — Stability Across Systems

Energy, Mood, Immunity Alignment

Energy production, mood regulation, and immune behavior operate as a coordinated system rather than independent outputs, and their alignment depends on the stability of redox conditions maintained by glutathione. Each of these domains draws from the same underlying resources, including mitochondrial output, substrate availability, and signaling balance. When glutathione capacity is sufficient, these systems operate in parallel with minimal interference. When it is limited, instability in one domain propagates into the others, creating a coupled pattern of dysfunction.

Energy production establishes the baseline for all other activity. Mitochondria generate ATP through electron transport, a process that inherently produces reactive intermediates. Glutathione contains these intermediates so that energy production can proceed without structural damage to the mitochondrial membrane or disruption of electron flow. When containment is effective, ATP production remains stable and predictable. When it is not, reactive accumulation alters membrane properties, increases electron leakage, and reduces efficiency, leading to fluctuating energy output.

Mood regulation depends on both energy availability and redox control within neural tissue. Neurotransmitter synthesis, release, and reuptake require consistent ATP supply, while signaling pathways depend on controlled redox conditions to maintain receptor function and intracellular communication. When glutathione maintains these conditions, signaling remains proportional and stable. When oxidative pressure increases, signaling becomes less controlled, receptor behavior shifts, and neurotransmitter balance becomes inconsistent. The result is variability in mood that reflects underlying instability rather than isolated changes in signaling molecules.

Immune activity competes for the same energy and redox resources. Activation increases metabolic demand and produces additional reactive intermediates that must be managed. When glutathione capacity is sufficient, immune responses can be initiated and resolved without disrupting energy production or neural signaling. When capacity is limited, immune activation diverts resources away from other systems, increasing oxidative load and reducing energy availability for non-immune processes. This creates a state where immune activity remains elevated while energy and mood stability decline.

The interaction between these systems becomes more apparent under sustained demand. Reduced energy output limits the ability of cells to maintain redox balance and complete repair processes. Persistent immune activation increases reactive production and further depletes glutathione. Neural signaling becomes less stable as both energy and redox conditions fluctuate. Each system amplifies the instability of the others, creating a reinforcing cycle rather than isolated dysfunction.

Alignment is restored when glutathione capacity supports stable redox conditions across all three domains. Energy production remains efficient, providing consistent ATP supply. Neural signaling operates within controlled parameters, maintaining stable mood and cognitive function. Immune responses activate when required and resolve without persistence. This alignment does not require maximizing any single system but maintaining balance so that none operates at the expense of the others.

Energy, mood, and immunity therefore reflect different expressions of the same underlying state. Glutathione determines whether that state is stable or unstable by controlling how reactive processes are contained and resolved. When capacity is sufficient, these systems remain coordinated and responsive. When it is reduced, they diverge and compete, producing variability that reflects a shared constraint rather than separate failures.

Chapter 31

Long-Term Resilience

Long-term resilience is the capacity of the system to maintain function across repeated cycles of demand without progressive loss of structure or control. It is not defined by the absence of stress or reactive processes, but by the ability to absorb those processes, resolve them completely, and return to baseline without accumulating residual damage. Glutathione sits at the center of this capacity because it determines whether redox balance can be restored after each cycle and whether structural components are preserved over time.

Resilience depends on maintaining a stable glutathione pool that can expand and contract in response to demand without becoming depleted. This requires continuous synthesis supported by consistent substrate availability, efficient recycling that preserves the active fraction of the pool, and controlled demand that does not exceed system capacity. When these elements are aligned, each cycle of oxidative activity is contained and resolved within its own timeframe. The system resets fully before the next cycle begins, preventing overlap and accumulation.

Structural preservation is a defining feature of resilience. Membranes retain their composition, proteins maintain functional configuration, and DNA remains intact across repeated exposures to reactive intermediates. Glutathione contributes to this preservation by limiting the propagation of reactions that would otherwise alter these structures. When protection is sufficient, normal maintenance processes can keep pace with minor alterations, replacing or repairing components without increasing overall system load.

Energy stability supports resilience by providing the consistent ATP supply required for synthesis, repair, and recycling. Mitochondrial function must remain efficient so that energy production does not generate excessive reactive intermediates while still meeting demand. When energy output is stable, the system can allocate resources to maintenance and recovery without compromising other functions. When it is unstable, repair processes slow, and incomplete resolution begins to accumulate.

Adaptation over time reflects the system's ability to adjust capacity based on repeated exposure to demand. When glutathione synthesis and recycling are responsive, the system can increase its baseline capacity to handle higher levels of activity without entering depletion. This adaptation is not a passive process. It requires that each cycle is completed successfully so that the system can build from a stable baseline rather than compensating for unresolved deficits.

Distribution across compartments is required for resilience at the system level. Each cellular compartment must maintain its own capacity to manage reactive processes. If one compartment becomes limited, localized damage accumulates and can propagate to other areas, reducing overall system stability. Coordinated availability across cytosol, mitochondria, and nucleus ensures that resilience is maintained uniformly rather than concentrated in a single pool.

Long-term resilience therefore reflects a system that can process demand repeatedly without degradation of function. It is built from continuous alignment between synthesis, recycling, energy production, and demand control. Glutathione enables this alignment by maintaining redox balance and supporting structural preservation. When this capacity is in place, the system remains stable over time, absorbing variability without accumulating damage and maintaining consistent performance across conditions.

Maintaining Glutathione Under Modern Stress

Maintaining glutathione under modern conditions requires sustaining continuous throughput in a system that is exposed to persistent, overlapping sources of demand. Reactive intermediates are generated at a higher baseline rate due to constant metabolic activity, environmental inputs, and repeated activation of detoxification and immune pathways. The system is not given extended periods of low demand where recovery can occur passively. Instead, it must operate in a state where synthesis, recycling, and utilization are active at all times. Stability depends on whether these processes can remain aligned under continuous load.

The primary challenge is maintaining a glutathione pool that does not collapse under sustained consumption. This requires uninterrupted substrate availability so that synthesis can proceed without gaps. Cysteine must be generated or delivered consistently, and glycine must remain available despite competing demands from repair and structural processes. Intermittent supply creates fluctuations in production that are amplified under constant demand, leading to periods where reactive intermediates are not contained immediately and system load increases.

Recycling must operate as a continuous process rather than a response to depletion. NADPH generation must match ongoing oxidation so that glutathione is returned to its reduced form as quickly as it is used. Under modern stress, this requirement becomes more pronounced because the rate of oxidation is elevated. If NADPH production fluctuates or declines, oxidized glutathione accumulates and reduces the effective capacity of the system even if total levels appear unchanged.

Demand control becomes a central factor because persistent exposure to reactive inputs increases consumption beyond what synthesis and recycling can sustain. Environmental compounds requiring detoxification, repeated immune activation, and unstable energy production all contribute to this demand. Lowering the rate at which glutathione is consumed allows the system to maintain a higher proportion of its pool in an active state, reducing the need for constant replacement and preventing progressive depletion.

Membrane composition influences how modern stress translates into system load. When membranes support controlled propagation of reactive events, the impact of each initiation is contained. When membranes are more susceptible, each event expands into multiple reactions, increasing demand on glutathione. Maintaining membrane structure that limits propagation reduces the total number of interactions that must be managed under continuous exposure.

Energy stability is required to sustain all supporting processes. ATP production must remain consistent so that synthesis can proceed and repair mechanisms can function without interruption. At the same time, metabolic pathways that generate NADPH must operate continuously to support recycling. Fluctuations in energy output create interruptions in both production and renewal, increasing the likelihood of depletion under sustained demand.

Maintaining glutathione under modern stress therefore requires the system to function as a continuous process rather than a reactive one. Substrate supply, enzymatic activity, recycling capacity, and demand control must all remain aligned over time. When this alignment is maintained, the system can operate under persistent load without progressive loss of capacity. When it is not, small imbalances accumulate, leading to gradual depletion and reduced ability to manage ongoing stress.

EPILOGUE

The Return of Order

Order returns to the system when processes that were operating in isolation are brought back into alignment and allowed to complete without interruption. The shift is not defined by a sudden change in any single variable but by the restoration of continuity across synthesis, utilization, and recovery. Glutathione reflects this shift because it sits at the point where reactive processes are either contained and resolved or allowed to propagate. When its availability and recycling are sufficient, reactions close, intermediates are cleared, and the system returns to a stable baseline before the next cycle begins.

The transition is measurable in how the system handles demand. Reactive intermediates are still generated, detoxification still occurs, and immune responses still activate, but each process now resolves within its intended timeframe. There is no carryover from one cycle to the next. Membranes retain their structure, proteins maintain function, and signaling remains proportional to input. The system no longer operates in a state of accumulation but in a state of controlled turnover where each event is completed and cleared.

Energy production stabilizes as mitochondrial function is no longer disrupted by persistent oxidative interference. Electron flow proceeds with fewer losses, reducing the formation of reactive intermediates at the source. This lowers demand on glutathione while simultaneously providing the ATP required for synthesis and repair. The system begins to operate with less strain, and processes that were previously competing for limited resources regain coordination.

Detoxification regains its sequence from modification to clearance. Compounds are processed once and removed rather than partially transformed and recirculated. This reduces background load and prevents repeated consumption of glutathione for the same inputs. Immune activity follows a similar pattern, activating when required and resolving fully once the initiating signal is addressed. Signaling pathways shut down cleanly, and the system returns to baseline without persistent activation.

This return to order is not a static state. It is a condition where the system can move through cycles of activity without losing structural integrity or control. Glutathione remains central because it determines whether each cycle is completed or left open. When completion capacity is restored, the system maintains its own stability through continuous alignment rather than external intervention.

The result is a system that no longer operates in deficit. Inputs are processed, outputs are resolved, and resources are renewed at a rate that matches or exceeds demand. Glutathione is not elevated as an isolated metric but maintained as part of a balanced system that supports consistent function over time. Order is therefore the restoration of sequence and completion, where each process begins, progresses, and ends without leaving unresolved burden behind.

Health as the Ability to Complete Stress Responses

Health reflects whether the system can move through a stress response from initiation to resolution without leaving residual disruption behind. Every stressor, whether metabolic, environmental, or immune, triggers a sequence that increases activity, generates reactive intermediates, and alters cellular conditions to address the input. This sequence is designed to be temporary. It begins with activation, progresses through processing, and ends with restoration of baseline conditions. Completion is the defining feature. When each stage proceeds without interruption, the system returns to its original state with structure and function preserved.

The ability to complete this sequence depends on maintaining sufficient glutathione to control reactive processes as they unfold. During activation, reactive intermediates are generated as part of signaling and defense. These intermediates must be neutralized after they have served their purpose, and glutathione provides the mechanism for that transition. If availability is sufficient and recycling is continuous, these signals are terminated within the same cycle, allowing the system to shift from an active state back to baseline without delay.

Failure to complete the response changes the behavior of the system. Reactive intermediates persist, signaling pathways remain active, and structural components are exposed to ongoing modification. Instead of a contained event, the system carries unresolved activity into the next cycle. This creates overlap where new stress responses begin before previous ones have been resolved, increasing total demand and reducing efficiency across all processes.

Energy production, detoxification, and immune signaling all depend on this completion. Energy systems must stabilize after increased output, detoxification pathways must carry compounds through to removal, and immune responses must shut down once their function is complete. Glutathione supports each of these transitions by restoring the redox conditions required for processes to end cleanly rather than persist.

Completion also preserves structural integrity over time. When stress responses are resolved fully, membranes retain their composition, proteins maintain function, and DNA remains protected from cumulative damage. When they are not, partial changes accumulate, altering system behavior and increasing vulnerability to subsequent stress.

Health therefore reflects the system's ability to process and resolve demand rather than avoid it. It is defined by continuity from activation through recovery, where each response is completed before the next begins. Glutathione determines whether this continuity is maintained by controlling how reactive processes are contained and resolved. When completion capacity is intact, the system remains stable across repeated exposures. When it is not, unresolved activity accumulates, and health declines as the system loses its ability to return to baseline.

Glutathione as a System Stabilizer, Not a Quick Fix

Glutathione stabilizes the system by maintaining the conditions required for processes to run to completion, rather than acting as an isolated intervention that produces immediate, visible effects. Its role is not to override dysfunction in a single step. It operates continuously within the background architecture, controlling how reactive intermediates are handled, how signals are terminated, and how structural components are preserved over time. When it is sufficient, the system maintains order across multiple domains without requiring constant correction.

A quick fix implies a direct input that produces a rapid and isolated outcome. Glutathione does not behave this way because its function is distributed across synthesis, recycling, and utilization. Increasing its availability at one point does not produce a stable effect if the rest of the system remains misaligned. Delivered glutathione is consumed within existing pathways, and any temporary increase is absorbed into ongoing turnover. Without supporting substrate flow, enzymatic activity, and demand control, the system returns to its prior state because the underlying structure has not changed.

Stabilization occurs when glutathione capacity is maintained at a level that allows each process to complete without leaving residual disruption. Reactive intermediates are neutralized within the same cycle in which they are generated, signaling pathways activate and shut down without persistence, and detoxification proceeds from modification to clearance without recirculation. These outcomes are not separate effects. They reflect a system that is operating with sufficient redox control to maintain continuity across processes.

The stabilizing role of glutathione is most visible in how it reduces variability. Energy production becomes consistent as mitochondrial function is no longer disrupted by uncontrolled reactive activity. Immune responses become proportional and self-limited rather than sustained. Neural signaling stabilizes as redox conditions support predictable receptor and neurotransmitter behavior. These changes emerge from the same underlying shift, where reactive processes are contained and resolved rather than allowed to accumulate.

This function requires continuous support rather than intermittent intervention. Substrates must be available for ongoing synthesis, recycling must restore oxidized glutathione as quickly as it is used, and demand must remain within the system's capacity to process. When these elements are aligned, glutathione maintains a steady-state presence that supports stability across conditions. When they are not, attempts to increase levels produce short-lived changes that do not persist.

Glutathione therefore acts as a stabilizer by preserving the conditions under which the system can regulate itself. It does not replace the need for coordinated function across pathways but enables that coordination by maintaining redox balance. When its capacity is sufficient, the system operates with continuity and control. When it is not, instability appears across multiple domains, reflecting the loss of a central mechanism that maintains order rather than a single deficiency that can be corrected in isolation.

Made in the USA
Monee, IL
05 November 2026

67914364R00134